AIDS LAW

IN A NUTSHELL

SECOND EDITION

By

ROBERT M. JARVIS
Professor of Law
Nova Southeastern University

MICHAEL L. CLOSEN
Professor of Law
John Marshall Law School

DONALD H.J. HERMANN
Professor of Law and Philosophy
Director, Health Law Institute
DePaul University College of Law

ARTHUR S. LEONARD
Professor of Law
New York Law School

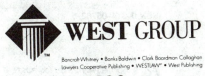

WEST GROUP

Bancroft-Whitney • Banks-Baldwin • Clark Boardman Callaghan
Lawyers Cooperative Publishing • WESTLAW • West Publishing

1996

COPYRIGHT © 1991 WEST PUBLISHING CO.
COPYRIGHT © 1996 By WEST PUBLISHING CO.
                    610 Opperman Drive
                    P.O. Box 64526
                    St. Paul, MN 55164–0526
                    1–800–328–9352

Library of Congress Cataloging-in-Publication Data

ISBN 0–314–06782–5

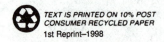

To those who help
those with AIDS

*

III

PREFACE
TO THE SECOND EDITION

Authors normally are delighted to be asked by their publishers to write a second edition. Not us. When we wrote the first edition of *AIDS Law in a Nutshell*, we hoped that the epidemic would be short lived and that there would be no need for a second edition of this book. Unfortunately, not only has the crisis not disappeared, it has grown worse. And while there have been small victories, such as Magic Johnson's recent return to the NBA, they have been overshadowed by the knowledge that the number of persons with HIV continues to increase daily.

As was true of the first edition of the Nutshell, we have sought to present, in short and readable fashion, the broad outlines of the law's response to the AIDS crisis. As will be seen, however, the organization of this new edition has changed considerably from that of the first edition. In part this is due to the need to conform to the structure of the second edition of our AIDS casebook, now known as *AIDS Law and Policy: Cases and Materials*, published by the John Marshall Publishing Company. The change also has been caused by the need to accommodate the numerous statutory and judicial developments that have occurred since publication of the first edition of the Nutshell in 1991. As a result, we have reformulated several of the chapters, relocated the discussion of various matters, and sought to place greater emphasis on the practical aspects of the subject at hand.

As before, we are most appreciative to our students and to the West Publishing Company. We also are grateful to the readers of the first edition of the Nutshell for their enthusiastic support, and hope that they deem this new edition a worthy effort.

ROBERT M. JARVIS
MICHAEL L. CLOSEN
DONALD H.J. HERMANN
ARTHUR S. LEONARD

Fort Lauderdale, FL
Chicago, IL
New York, NY
March 1996

PREFACE
TO THE FIRST EDITION

It now has been ten years since AIDS was first discovered. In some ways, ten years is a very long time, while in others it is just a passing moment in history. These past ten years have been a remarkable time, filled with much despair and agony at the loss of thousands of individuals to a new and horrible disease, yet infused with a sense of hope and wonder as medicine has pushed back the frontiers of science with awe-inspiring speed. It has, to paraphrase another, been the best of times and the worst of times.

AIDS has had an enormous impact on the legal system as the problems faced by people with AIDS have come to touch every aspect of society and its activities. AIDS-specific laws have been passed in many jurisdictions, numerous lawsuits involving AIDS have been filed (and decided), and AIDS has come to influence every level of government thinking and action. Many law schools now offer a course on AIDS, and it is no longer possible to count the number of treatises, symposia, and law review and bar journal articles on AIDS.

Thus, after a decade of experience with AIDS, it seems that the time is right for a nutshell on what now is beginning to be recognized as a specialized field of its own. AIDS law is, of course, a collection of many older fields of law—such as criminal law, family law, and insurance law—and it remains a branch of health law. But it seems to us that AIDS law also can be meaningfully discussed and thought of as a field that is charting its own separate path. Indeed, we are beginning to witness the advent of lawyers who spend most of their professional time engaged with the problems of persons with AIDS.

Every book has its beginning, and this book is no exception. The idea for this book was born in the summer of 1989, just after the authors, together with others, had put the finishing touches on a law school casebook entitled *AIDS: Cases and Materials* (John Marshall Publishing Company 1989). Reflecting on the vast amount of material contained in that book, it became apparent to us that there was a need for a primer that law students could turn to for ready guidance on the legal aspects of the AIDS epidemic. Further discussion convinced us that such a work also might be helpful to practitioners as well as to those in the medical arts and the public at large. When the West Publishing Company agreed, this book began to become a reality.

Because this book is intended to be read and used by a number of different audiences, some of whom may be unfamiliar with law, we have attempted to keep the number of statutory and case references to a minimum and to avoid the use of typical legal jargon. For those readers who are using this book in conjunction with *AIDS: Cases and Materials,* a word needs to be said about the organization of this book. Although this book is intended to supplement the casebook, certain organizational changes have been made. Thus, Chapters 2 and 3 of the case-book are covered in Chapter 2 of this book, Chapters 7 and 8 of the casebook are treated as Chapter 6 of this book, and Chapters 14 and 15 of the casebook are discussed in Chapter 12 of this book. As a result, with the exception of Chapter 1, the numbering system of this book does not correspond directly to the numbering system of the casebook.

As with any writing project, we are indebted to a number of individuals who helped in the production of this book. We are especially appreciative of the efforts of the West Publishing Company, which believed in our idea and helped us with all phases of the production process. We also would like to thank Leslie Deckelbaum and Lillian Sartell. They provided timely and efficient typing and word processing assistance and without them this book would not have been completed. Finally, we are indebted to all of the students in our respective AIDS courses. They have taught us as much about this area of the law as we have taught them.

ROBERT M. JARVIS
MICHAEL L. CLOSEN
DONALD H.J. HERMANN
ARTHUR S. LEONARD

Fort Lauderdale, FL
Chicago, IL
New York, NY
July 1990

*

OUTLINE

_____

OUTLINE

*

TABLE OF CASES

References are to Pages

TABLE OF CASES

TABLE OF CASES

*

AIDS LAW

IN A NUTSHELL

SECOND EDITION

*

CHAPTER I

OVERVIEW

A. INTRODUCTION

Taken as a whole, have the responses of the medical, business, governmental, legal, and political communities to AIDS differed from society's responses to other diseases throughout history? Probably not very much. At least one appellate court, for instance, has referred to AIDS as "the modern day equivalent of leprosy." *South Florida Blood Service, Inc. v. Rasmussen.*

Many people naively think of disease or health concerns as purely objective, and certainly mumps, measles, and the common cold tend to be fairly objective in nature. Yet numerous other diseases have occupied less than glorious moments in history. Even the reactions to people afflicted with cancer and tuberculosis have been less than exemplary at times—not to mention the discrimination directed at people with leprosy, syphilis, herpes, hepatitis, and other dreaded conditions.

For those who wish to find similarities between AIDS and other infectious diseases, there are several candidates for comparison. AIDS is caused by a virus, and so are herpes, smallpox, yellow fever, and hepatitis. AIDS is fatal, and yellow fever, plague,

1

smallpox, and Legionnaire's disease also can be deadly. Symptoms and severe illness due to AIDS may develop over extended periods of time, and this is the same with leprosy, tuberculosis, and syphilis. AIDS can be terribly disfiguring and horrifying, and so can smallpox and leprosy. AIDS often is associated with unpopular groups (gay men and intravenous drug users), and so are hepatitis B (gay men) and syphilis (promiscuous individuals).

It often is said that history tends to repeat itself. The AIDS era seems to be no exception. Perhaps more than any other disease in history, AIDS has been politicized. Many reasons account for this development. One is the time at which AIDS was identified—the early 1980s. It was a time just after a conservative Republican president (Ronald Reagan) had taken office. The groups most affected—gay men and intravenous drug users—were unpopular. Another minority group—African-Americans—was labeled by some as the source of AIDS because it was thought that the disease may have originated in Africa. Some of the modes of transmission of AIDS—anonymous and near-anonymous sex and intravenous drug use—are disfavored. Other important factors include the disease's elusive and seemingly incurable nature, its gruesome and fatal consequences, and its exorbitant costs.

Unwarranted discrimination against persons with AIDS, against persons perceived to have AIDS, and against persons though to be at heightened risk for AIDS, has been widespread. Some individuals have lost their jobs, their insurance protection, their access to public education, and their ability to visit friends or family. Others have been refused medical treatment, nursing home care, housing, and funeral services. Still others have been forced to submit to testing. These examples constitute only a small glimpse of the many areas of concern for people with AIDS, people suspected of having AIDS, and people believed to be at increased risk of contracting AIDS.

AIDS has humbled many in the medical and scientific communities, has led others to doubt the genuineness of governmental and medical efforts to treat and cure the disease, and has caused a wide range of negative emotions, including depression, frustration, pain, hysteria, and even suicide. Before AIDS, it seemed as though science could conquer just about any health problem. Polio, tuberculosis, some forms of cancer, syphilis, and Legionnaire's disease all had been tamed through advances in medical knowledge. But neither a vaccine nor a cure for AIDS is expected any time soon.

Although AIDS began as a medical problem, it is today a legal problem of enormous dimensions. As has been written elsewhere:

Because the epidemic is growing and a cure is not yet in sight, AIDS creates pressures on all aspects of law and the legal system. Legislatures and public health authorities are responding to the disease by adopting provisions that deal specifically with HIV infection. The growing body of

law that tests the validity of this special legislation and rulemaking is likely to have substantial
impact on all aspects of health care and health
care law long after the AIDS epidemic has passed.

M. Hall & I. Ellman, *Health Care Law and Ethics
in a Nutshell* 389 (1990).

B. MEDICAL BACKGROUND

Although there now is competent retrospective
evidence that Acquired Immune Deficiency Syndrome (AIDS) has afflicted mankind since at least
the 1950s, the disease was not recognized as a
unique condition until 1981. The identification of
AIDS was accidental, and occurred when a few
doctors began to notice small clusters of cases of
highly unusual and fatal opportunistic infections in
young, otherwise healthy men in New York City
and San Francisco. The two infections that attacked these men were Kaposi's Sarcoma (KS) and
Pneumocystis Carinii Pneumonia (PCP). Although
KS and PCP remain hallmark indicators for an
AIDS diagnosis, other symptoms and serologic testing now make it possible to recognize AIDS in
patients who do not have either KS or PCP.

Doctors and health authorities accumulating information on the early cases quickly noticed that
the patients shared a number of common factors:
1) they were sexually active gay men, 2) they lived
in either New York City or San Francisco, and, 3)
they had suppressed immune systems that were
susceptible to KS and PCP. As more cases arose, it

was noted that some of the men with AIDS used recreational stimulants, including intravenous drugs, while others were of Haitian origin. Later, as still more cases were reported, women, blood transfusion patients, and intravenous drug users were found to have AIDS. Newborn babies, recipients of blood products and organ and tissue donations, and sexually active heterosexual and bisexual individuals also were diagnosed as having AIDS. Eventually, it was determined that AIDS was caused by a virus called lymphadenopathy-associated virus (LAV) by some and human T-cell lymphotropic virus type III (HTLV–III) by others. The virus later was renamed the Human Immunodeficiency Virus (HIV) and a blood test was developed and marketed to identify antibodies to the virus.

People who die as a result of the disease condition now known as AIDS do not actually die of AIDS itself. Rather, they die from one or more of the opportunistic infections that afflict people with AIDS. The reason that these opportunistic infections kill is that HIV causes a person's immune system to become suppressed or ineffective in performing its primary role in the body, namely, the fighting of disease and infections.

HIV invades certain key blood cells (known as T-cells) and replicates, spreads, and destroys the host cells along the way. HIV has now been found throughout the bodies of HIV-infected individuals in every body fluid and even in the brain. Thus, infections that ordinarily would be prevented or fought by the body's immune system in individuals who do not have HIV become deadly in people with HIV.

1. Incidence

More than 40,000 new cases of AIDS are reported each year in the United States, and it is estimated that 500,000 Americans have been dignosed as having AIDS since the start of the epidemic in 1981. Of this number, a total of 311,000 people—or 62%— have already died.

Some 50,000 cases of AIDS were reported during the period 1981–87.   Over the next four years (1988–92), 205,000 new cases were reported. Between 1993 and 1995, 245,000 additional cases were found.   Although drawing comparisons among these three time periods is somewhat difficult because the definition of AIDS was changed after 1992 to take into account symptoms that are chiefly experienced by women, and because there is no uniform requirement to report positive HIV tests to public health officials, the explosion in the prevalence of AIDS in the United States is indisputable.

AIDS first appeared in the United States in the Northeast and the West, and rates remain highest in the Northeast.   The greatest proportionate increases, however, are now taking place in the Midwest and the South, due in large part to infections among adolescents and young adults in rural areas and small cities. The leading origin of infection in the South is heterosexual activity, while in the Midwest it is drug use. Nationally, however, drug use (27%, up from 17% in the early years of the epidemic) is by far a much more important means of transmission than heterosexual sex (10%, up from 3% in 1987). At the same time, HIV transmission through homosexual intercourse has dropped to less than 50% of all new cases.

AIDS is primarily a disease of the young (including newborn infants): one out of every four new cases of HIV infection occurs among Americans under the age of 20 and HIV-related illnesses are the leading cause of death among adults between the ages of 25 and 44. Besides the young, certain sub-populations in the United States suffer from HIV and AIDS in much larger numbers than the population as a whole. The incidence of AIDS is six times greater for African–Americans than it is for whites. For Hispanic–Americans, the figure is three times larger than for whites. African–Americans now account for 38%, and Hispanic–Americans for 18%, of the total number of AIDS cases in the United States.

The number of women who are HIV-positive is also growing at an alarming rate. Whereas women once accounted for only a handful of new AIDS cases, they now make up 18% of all such cases. African–American women are particularly vulnerable; it has been estimated, for example, that such a woman is fifteen times more likely than a white woman to be HIV-positive.

Although AIDS cuts across social, economic, racial, and sexual lines, the media has tended to focus on celebrities who are either HIV-positive or have died of AIDS. Famous personalities who have contracted the disease include Rock Hudson, Arthur Ashe, Liberace, Perry Ellis, Freddie Mercury, Greg Louganis, Anthony Perkins, Michael Bennett, Halston, Robert Reed, Roy Cohn, and Denholm Elliott.

No celebrity with HIV has been watched more closely than Earvin "Magic" Johnson, the popular former captain of the Los Angeles Lakers. Forced to retire from the National Basketball Association in November 1991 after discovering that he was HIV-positive, Johnson made a triumphant return to the league in February 1996 (but retired again in May 1996). Many observers believe that Johnson's return signals a new acceptance on the part of society towards people with HIV and AIDS. Even as Johnson was resuming his career, however, President Clinton was signing legislation (which was later repealed) that required the military to discharge anyone testing positive for HIV.

2. Modes of Transmission

It has been determined that HIV can be transmitted in a small number of very specific ways, namely, by the exchange from person to person of certain kinds of bodily fluids (but not all bodily fluids). Thus, HIV can be contracted by:

(a) Sexual intercourse through the exchange of blood, semen, and vaginal secretions. Receptive anal intercourse is the highest risk activity for sexual transmission of HIV due to the possibility that during the vigor of intercourse tiny tears or breaks in the lining of the rectum will result and allow blood or semen from the other individual to enter the system of the receptive partner. For similar reasons, receptive vaginal intercourse is also a risky activity for the transmission of HIV.

(b) Sharing the unsterilized syringes used in intravenous drug injections, due to the exchange of infected blood.

(c) Receipt of donations of blood, semen, breast milk, organs, and other human tissue.

(d) Child birth or breastfeeding of a newborn (transmission vertically from mother to child).

(e) Possibly as the result of invasive medical procedures, such as surgeries or dental extractions of teeth. It has been documented that six patients of an HIV-infected Florida dentist named David Acer (including Kimberly Bergalis, who later became a national spokeswoman for the testing of health care workers) somehow contracted HIV. But it is not known whether the transmissions were intentional or accidental. Thousands of patients who have undergone invasive care by other HIV-infected doctors and dentists have been examined and have been found not to be infected.

One of the parties to the activities listed above must be HIV-infected in order to transmit the virus to the other party; importantly, casual contact does not transmit HIV. Hence, if an uninfected person shakes hands with, hugs, shares eating utensils with, kisses, or sits on a toilet seat after someone with AIDS, the virus will not be transmitted.

3. Theories of Origin

When AIDS was first recognized, it was quite natural that doctors, researchers, governmental health officials, and others concerned about the possible spread of a new disease began to identify groups at risk for AIDS. At first, AIDS was thought to be almost entirely a disease of homosexual men because the first cases that were reported involved gays. Soon, however, some people from the country of Haiti began to experience the disease and intravenous drug users also were identified as having AIDS. All of this explains, in substantial part, why there was such discrimination, panic, and hysteria about AIDS in the early years after its discovery. It was a deadly condition. It was incurable. It was spread by activities that were not well thought of in many segments of the population—namely, sex and drugs. The people who suffered from AIDS were unpopular: gay men, drug users, and immigrants from a Caribbean island.

As time went on, recipients of blood components (hemophiliacs) and whole blood (blood transfusion recipients) started to fall prey to AIDS and newborn babies were discovered with AIDS. Bisexual men, male and female prostitutes, and other individuals also were found to have AIDS. Today, the profile of who is at increased risk of contracting AIDS has changed significantly from the first days of the epidemic. Because HIV entered the general population through the blood supply and through sexual intercourse, every segment of the population has suffered some level of AIDS.

It is understandable that the question of the origin of AIDS was raised very early. Perhaps it was due somewhat to idle curiosity. Certainly it was due in part to the epidemiological efforts of medical researchers to find ways to treat and cure AIDS. While some of the theories of the origin of AIDS are founded upon reason, others are rooted in ignorance, hysteria, and prejudice. A few of the theories do serve to explain in part the reason for the spread of AIDS, but they do not identify the source of the disease. Listed below are several of the better-known theories of the origin of AIDS.

(a) *Patient Zero Theory.* Very early in the epidemic, when it was still possible to keep close track of all of the reported cases of AIDS, researchers discovered a common link in approximately forty individuals with AIDS. That link was a young gay man named Gaetan Dugas who worked as a flight attendant for Air Canada and who was infected with HIV. He traveled around the world and engaged in sex with numerous partners. Many of them got AIDS and eventually he did too. We now know that Dugas could not have been the very first person with AIDS. Retrospective evidence demonstrates that AIDS was present prior to Dugas. Furthermore, even if he was "Patient Zero," we still would not know how Dugas got AIDS. However, the research regarding him supports the propositions that sex with multiple partners and international mobility do contribute to the spread of AIDS.

(b) *God's Retribution Theory (or Sexual Practice Theory).* The retribution theory is the much-preached theory that AIDS is God's punishment against gay men and intravenous drug users for their alleged violations of the laws of nature and man. There seems to be an unfortunate side of human nature that needs to find blame for anything that cannot be readily explained or understood. Disease, especially one that can be spread by sex or by the use of some types of addictive drugs, cannot remain merely objective. People need to scapegoat and attach blame. The advocates of the retribution theory, however, cannot explain why blood transfusion recipients, children, and others should be punished by contracting AIDS. The advocates of this theory only make a tragic situation more tragic. They contribute to the ignorance and hysteria that have impeded progress in coping with AIDS.

(c) *Biological Warfare Theory.* A few people, thought to be rather extreme in their views, have proposed that AIDS is the result of research and testing aimed at developing weapons for biological and chemical warfare. The adherents to this theory are somewhat divided as to whether some germ or virus was accidentally created and escaped into the environment to pillage as it has, or whether the germ or virus was purposely unleashed into the gay and drug-using populations in the mistaken belief that it would remain confined to those groups. Other advocates of the biological warfare theory focus on the fact that AIDS may have received its start in the nations of Africa and that AIDS does affect people of color in this country in disproportionately high numbers. These advocates see AIDS as a racist plot. There seems to be no objective evidence whatsoever to support any of the claims that a manufactured virus or diabolical plan is at the root of AIDS. *Traufler v. Thompson.*

(d) *Co-Factor Theory.* A fairly popular theory among medical researchers and others holds that AIDS is the result of some combination of factors that, by happenstance, cause the suppression of the immune system. These co-factors are behavioral matters, such as a person's sexual practices, lifestyle, diet, use of drugs, and general health. It appears that it will never be possible to prove this theory. Now that AIDS has spread as widely as it has, seemingly every combination of co-factors is represented among those persons who have developed the disease.

(e) *Poppers Theory.* There was a brief period, very early in the history of AIDS, when some researchers advanced the poppers theory. In a number of the initial cases, doctors discovered that the patient had used an inhalant stimulant known as amil nitrate, or poppers. Thus, it was thought that the use of poppers, either alone or in conjunction with some other co-factor, was the cause of AIDS. This theory was proved incorrect, however, when it was shown that many young people were inhaling poppers without getting AIDS. It was simply a component of many of the first individuals who developed AIDS. Nevertheless, the advocates of the poppers theory did identify a very significant, albeit indirect, reason for the spread of AIDS. Since the use of substances such as alcohol and drugs tends to diminish inhibitions and, as a result, can lead to an increased willingness to engage in sexual intercourse and intravenous drug use, the poppers theory's emphasis on lifestyle as a factor in predicting who is at risk of contracting AIDS is accurate.

(f) *Mutation Theory (or Primate Theory)*. A substantial number of knowledgeable people from both the medical and scientific fields believe that HIV originated as a mutation from some virus that afflicted another animal species (thus the reason why this theory also has been referred to as the primate or simian theory of the origin of AIDS). There are similarities between AIDS and diseases in cats and monkeys, and body parts of monkeys were used in the research and cultivation of the polio vaccine. There also was extensive testing of the vaccine in Africa. Perhaps that was the jumping-off point for AIDS.

It is well known that HIV is not a simple virus but a number of variations on a virus that is subject to frequent mutation. This constant variation in the virus complicates the efforts of medical science to discover ways to treat and prevent infection. Indeed, it has been posited that if AIDS originated as a mutation from some other virus in another species, we may have to await another mutation that will fortuitously render AIDS non-deadly or will cause the virus to disappear naturally (and in either case free society from its grip).

4. Development of Symptoms

After an individual is exposed to HIV through one of the recognized modes of transmission, the individual may or may not become infected with HIV. Why this is so remains a mystery, just as it is unclear why some people will catch the common cold in the same circumstances in which others do not. Once an individual is infected with HIV, it takes the body a certain amount of time to undergo a sufficient immune system reaction to develop antibodies.

There is a period of time when a person who is infected with HIV will not test positive on a HIV antibody test. This "window" period lasts somewhere between three weeks and six months in 95% of infected persons, although a few researchers have suggested that the window period may last several years in some individuals.

After infection, an individual will be asymptomatic for a period of time. During this period many persons suffer a short encounter with minor and generalized symptoms that constitute their initial reaction to HIV. This early experience will almost never be recognized as the beginning of HIV infection, for it is too short and too generalized. Hence, it is usually attributed to a simple bout of the common cold, the flu, or fatigue.

An HIV-infected individual usually remains asymptomatic for a very long period of time. Most experts now place this period of time, on average, between five and ten years. Thereafter, one or more symptoms will begin to appear. In the early days of the epidemic, these symptoms were referred to as ARC (for AIDS–Related Complex). That terminology has now been largely abandoned.

As individuals progress from the asymptomatic stage of HIV disease to full-blown AIDS, a number of symptoms have become well-recognized as indicators of the failing of the immune system. It should be emphasized that not all individuals with HIV will experience all of these symptoms—some people will suffer from one or two of the conditions while others will show several of the symptoms. It also should be emphasized that unless the symptoms listed below are profound or serious and long-term in nature, they should not necessarily be regarded as suggestive of AIDS. Furthermore, in order to be indicative of AIDS these symptoms must not be explainable in any other way (such as being the result of dieting, anemia, or other health problems). The classic symptoms of AIDS include:

(a) A general swelling of the lymph nodes, particularly around the neck and chin, the armpits, and the groin, with enlargement that does not subside. This condition is referred to as lymphadenopathy.

(b) Loss of 10% or more of one's body weight over a relatively short period of time. AIDS is often referred to in Africa as "slim disease" due to the emaciated condition of many of its victims.

(c) Profound fatigue which is so severe that one feels unable to get out of bed and move about (causing some individuals to sleep 15 to 20 hours a day).

(d) Profuse sweating at night that leaves one's bedding entirely soaked and requires a number of changes during the night.

(e) Extensive and long-lasting oral thrush characterized by white spots or areas in the mouth and throat that do not rinse or brush away.

(f) Prolonged low-grade fever lasting for weeks at a time that fails to respond to aspirin or similar therapies.

(g) Diarrhea and other intestinal and bowel irregularities that continue for many days or weeks at a time.

(h) Persistent skin irritations on various parts of the body.

Besides these generalized and very individualized symptoms, serious opportunistic diseases may attack the depressed immune systems of people with AIDS. Such ailments can include KS (signaled by blue-black lesions on the body), PCP (signaled by shortness of breath), tuberculosis, shingles, blindness, and dementia. Such opportunistic infections ultimately take the lives of persons with AIDS unless some intervening cause results in an even earlier death.

5. HIV Testing

In March 1985, a serologic test for the antibodies to HIV was marketed. Although this blood test is sometimes referred to as an "AIDS test," it is not really an AIDS test at all. It neither discovers the presence of the virus nor plays the exclusive diagnostic role of identifying AIDS. Instead, the HIV test detects the antibodies that are developed by the body's immune system in response to infection with HIV. An AIDS diagnosis requires both a positive HIV test result and a clinical identification of a recognized symptom of AIDS (such as a T-cell count of 200 or less, KS, or PCP).

The standard procedure for the completion of an HIV test is for a patient's blood to be drawn and labelled and then sent to a laboratory for a preliminary screening test known as the enzyme-linked immunoabsorbent assay (ELISA). Blood that appears positive for HIV antibodies is subjected to a second confirmatory test called the Western blot that may or may not show the sample to be positive for HIV antibodies. Finally, the test results are recorded and returned to the source that submitted the blood sample.

As with all forms of medical testing, HIV testing is not always accurate. There is room for human error in a number of ways. The blood sample may be improperly labeled or the test results might be inaccurately recorded. The administration of the test may be faulty or the evaluation of the results may be erroneously performed. Moreover, the test itself is not completely reliable, for there is a slight possibility of false positive and false negative results.

Because the ELISA is highly sensitive, many blood samples report HIV-positive or indeterminate when in fact they are not seropositive. The Western blot is a far more accurate tool for determining HIV antibody status, although its high cost rules out its use as an initial screening device. When properly administered and interpreted, the two-step test protocol is thought to be more than 99% accurate.

Importantly, as previously observed, there is a window period between the time one becomes infected with HIV and the time when the body's immune system has had enough of an opportunity to develop an antibody reaction sufficient to trigger a positive HIV test result. Individuals are particularly infectious during this window period. Thus, if people are tested while in the window period, the presence of HIV antibodies will not be detected even though such people are infected and infectious. This explains, in part, why the American blood supply is not completely safe even today, at a time when all blood donations are supposed to be screened for HIV. There remains a very slight possibility that HIV-infected blood can get into the blood supply system.

In the relatively near future, a new generation of AIDS tests will become widely available. Unlike previous tests, these new tests react directly to the presence of the virus, signifying not only its presence but also its quantity. Thus, doctors will be able to determine whether a person is infected quite soon after exposure, with the window period collapsed to just a few days. Equally important for treatment purposes, doctors will be able to monitor the level of the virus present in the body and adjust treatment strategies accordingly. Although these expensive new tests are not yet in general use, they will eventually supplant the less reliable antibody testing for a variety of purposes.

6. Treatment and Research

In the early 1980s, most individuals found to have the disease died rather soon after diagnoses of AIDS, usually of a single opportunistic infection (most often PCP). A number of reasons explain this perceived rapid course to death. First, because it was not then understood that there was a long period of time between infection with HIV and the development of symptoms, the thought prevailed that infection must rapidly lead to death. Second, because there was no blood test for HIV antibodies and because few physicians were well informed about AIDS, people were identified as having AIDS only when they were far along in the course of their disease. Third, because the early symptoms of AIDS are so generalized and individualized that they may signal any number of health problems, many cases of AIDS went unrecognized until very late in the progression towards death.

Over time, medical science has made considerable progress in diagnosing AIDS. The advent of antibody testing allowed for earlier detection of infected individuals. Additionally, medical science has had marked success in treating a number of the opportunistic infections associated with AIDS. By the late 1980s, the FDA had licensed Azovidine (AZT), a drug that appeared to prolong the period between infection and development of symptomatic AIDS by slowing the ability of HIV to replicate in the body. By the early 1990s, use of AZT, frequently in combination with other drugs, became the state-of-the-art treatment, although continuing mutation of the virus within a patient's body meant that even combination therapies lost their effectiveness over time as the virus developed resistance to the medication.

In the mid-1990s, research progressed to a new generation of AIDS drugs, called protease inhibitors, which seemed much more powerful in preventing viral replication. Strategic use of these drugs, in combination with a new generation of HIV tests to monitor "viral load" (the volume of virus present in the blood), theoretically gave physicians the tools to make AIDS a more manageable condition with longer survival times. However, both the new drugs and the new tests are significantly more expensive than earlier treatments, prompting debate about how widespread their use could become.

Research to develop a vaccine that might confer immunity to HIV infection began with isolation of the virus in the mid-1980s but had not borne fruit over its first decade. HIV is a virus that reproduces quickly, with each cycle generating mutations in the proteins of its surface coating. Traditional vaccine theories depend upon stimulating an immune response through the introduction of harmless matter that simulates the targeted pathogen (such as killed virus or a compound made from bits of the viral coating), thus preparing the body with a ready template for quick antibody production if the actual pathogen later appears. Such a strategy is difficult to pursue with a rapidly mutating virus such as HIV.

In addition, current theories on how HIV causes AIDS indicate that the problem is not the body's failure to form antibodies, but rather that HIV seems to outrun the body's capabilities as it continues mutating and replicating while the body constantly goes back to square one to make new antibodies. Preparing the body with a first set of antibodies, even if one could anticipate which precise strain of the virus was likely to be the invader, might only be a stopgap measure unless a way is found to insure that the initial antibody supply could totally eliminate the invader, thus cutting off its ability to mutate in the body.

Before drugs and other treatment therapies can be used by physicians and paid for under government programs, they must be licensed by the Food and Drug Administration (FDA). In addition, most private insurance plans will pay only for licensed drugs and treatments, explicitly excluding coverage for "experimental" treatments. By statute, the FDA must determine that drugs and other treatments are both safe and effective before licensing takes place. Prior to changes provoked by the AIDS epidemic, this process was complex, difficult, expensive, and time-consuming. Under normal pre-AIDS conditions, it took between eight and ten years for a new drug to win FDA approval.

Even before AIDS came along, there was controversy about the FDA's process of dealing with new drugs. Arguments were advanced that individuals with serious, life-threatening diseases for which there were no licensed effective treatments should be able to obtain access to experimental treatments that were not ready for licensure. Persons who claimed to suffer from terminal cancers went to court to gain access to laetrile, an untested cancer drug that was generally available in Mexico. In

United States v. Rutherford, the United States Supreme Court rejected their plea, reasoning that there could not be a prospective diagnosis of terminal cancer.

By the late 1980s, some AIDS treatment activists were mounting heavy pressure on the FDA (including highly publicized demonstrations and an occupation of the FDA's headquarters) to speed consideration of new AIDS treatments. Responding to pressure from activists, legislators, and government officials outside the normal drug review process, the FDA agreed to experiment with methods of speeding access, including authorizing larger scale "safety" testing of promising drugs in patient populations and relaxing enforcement of rules against individuals bringing unapproved drugs into the United States from other countries.

In a significant departure from past practices, the FDA also moved to involve primary care doctors in drug trials in which their patients were enlisted. Previously, all drug testing took place within highly controlled laboratory settings administered by research scientists. Community-based testing, by contrast, authorized the release of drugs whose safety had been relatively well-established but whose efficacy was still uncertain, to be administered to consenting patients of cooperating physicians, with the physicians pressed into the role of monitoring and reporting the results. Thus, the newest drugs, frequently provided at no charge due to their experimental nature, could be obtained by patients astute enough to seek out participating physicians or medical centers.

In addition to these officially sanctioned openings for unlicensed treatments, a substantial underground movement developed to provide such drugs to people with AIDS. Drugs approved in other countries but not in the United States have been smuggled into this country by operatives of buyer cooperatives. Drugs unapproved anywhere have been manufactured and circulated to some people with AIDS, and various homemade concoctions went in and out of favor as anecdotal evidence was shared through networks of patients and doctors. AIDS presented the unusual development of a substantial patient population attempting to supplant what was seen as a sluggish and non-responsive medical establishment in exploring new treatments. There is an ongoing debate about the wisdom, ethics, and legality of these actions.

7. Status as a Chronic Condition

Although this book frequently uses the term "AIDS" for purposes of simplicity, it is actually more accurate to speak about "HIV disease" or "HIV–AIDS." The consensus of medical authority is that a focus on AIDS (or what is sometimes referred to as full-blown AIDS) neglects the significant role of HIV infection as the precursor of AIDS and as a long-term health problem of its own with important implications for testing, prevention, and treatment.

The view that HIV and AIDS must be treated as separate health threats stems from a number of developments. Medical science has found that a long period of time may intervene between infection with HIV and development of the serious symptoms of AIDS. As noted earlier, this period can last for as long as ten or more years. Medical science also has become progressively more capable of delaying the onset of opportunistic infections and treating them when they occur, leading directly to an increase in life expectancy from the time of infection. The life span from time of infection may be twenty years or more for those with access to state-of-the-art treatment and some luck, and future medical advances may increase this. Because most of those infected are relatively young, this means that many people will be living for significant periods of time with AIDS as a chronic, managed condition.

Because HIV infection is often asymptomatic for years, people can be infected and infectious for substantial periods. This fact, of course, contributes to the spread of the disease. People with HIV can transmit the disease for a long time (whereas it once was thought that they fell seriously ill quickly and died). The long asymptomatic period can lead to a false sense of safety among some infected people, thereby contributing to a further transmission of the disease. Early voluntary testing can help detect seropositive individuals, who hopefully will act responsibly so as to avoid conduct that is known to risk transmission of HIV. In addition, early detection of HIV-infection is increasingly valuable to individuals as new treatments make it possible to delay the onset of full-blown AIDS.

With developments in some drug treatment therapies, early detection of HIV can contribute to substantially prolonged life (for those who decide to learn of their HIV condition and seek treatment). Thus, voluntary HIV testing is again a method to obtain early knowledge of the presence of HIV and in turn identify those who wish to promptly commence therapy.

8. Education and Prevention

Efforts to educate the public about AIDS in order to reduce the panic and hysteria about the disease and prevent its further spread are widely needed. To date, however, such efforts have been implemented only haphazardly.

Education about AIDS is needed in all classrooms at all levels of instruction. The content of the information needs to be thorough and sufficiently explicit to alert audiences to the modes of transmission and to the steps that can be taken to eliminate or reduce the possibility of transmission. Although abstinence from sex and drugs can be encouraged, instruction about safe sex and methods for sterilization of drug needles needs to be included and graphically described. References to sexual intercourse, including anal intercourse and the use of condoms, cannot be avoided for the sake of etiquette.

There also needs to be an expansive program of neighborhood and governmental outreach programs in shelters for the homeless and the needy and in other community facilities to reach the people of the street who engage in intravenous drug use, prostitution, promiscuous sex, or combinations of these activities. Again, the instruction needs to be interesting and graphic in order to hold the attention of the audience.

Three groups with the highest incidence of new HIV infections are women (particularly women of color), adolescents, and newborns. An important segment of the group of adolescents (who may or may not encounter AIDS education through the school system) and the people of the street are prospective mothers. Because of the staggering problems faced by newborn infants with HIV infection, much needs to be done to education prospective mothers, including the urging of voluntary anonymous HIV testing. Legislation enacted in 1996 predicates federal AIDS funding for states and localities on the development of effective counseling and voluntary testing programs for pregnant women. If significant reductions of the incidence of HIV-infected newborns are not achieved, the legislation mandates nonconsensual testing of newborns.

That HIV education can help to prevent transmission of the disease has been proven by the example of the organized gay community's educational programs in New York City, San Francisco, Los Angeles, Chicago, Miami, Houston, and other large cities. The gay community has succeeded in significantly reducing the rate of new transmissions and new infections with HIV (although there is evidence that the decline may not be permanent). In contrast, the numbers of new HIV infections among intravenous drug users, women, newborn children, and adolescents is increasing rapidly.

C. AIDS AND POLITICS

Almost from the moment when it was first discovered, AIDS has been a very political disease. While it may be open to debate whether AIDS has been politicized to a greater extent than past diseases, no one now questions (if they ever did) that every aspect of AIDS, including research, treatment, funding, and legislative initiatives, has been influenced to a remarkable degree by political considerations. It also is generally agreed that AIDS has become more political over time and that the future is likely to see politicization increase rather than subside.

1. Early Politicization

During the early years of the AIDS epidemic, most of the attention that was paid to AIDS came from conservative political groups and candidates and incumbents seeking the electoral support of such groups. Buoyed by the recent election of Ronald Reagan to the presidency of the United States, conservatives in the early 1980s believed that their time was at hand. They were determined to push forward a political agenda whose centerpiece was a return to traditional family values and a renewed emphasis on personal morality.

AIDS presented society with a disease that seemed to bear out everything that conservatives stood for and supported. As a disease primarily transmitted through homosexual intercourse and drug use, AIDS proved useful to conservatives in two ways. First, it buttressed the argument that the nation was suffering grievously from the excesses of the sexual revolution, the increased willingness to recognize and accord legitimacy to the gay lifestyle, and the greater tolerance towards and participation in recreational drugs. Second, it permitted homosexuals and drug users to be portrayed as loathsome, unclean, and deadly.

AIDS also helped conservatives in another way. Many of the earliest cases were reported among Haitian immigrants. As dark-skinned individuals who often spoke little or no English, worked at menial jobs, and remained on the fringe of society for fear of being detected by American immigration officials and sent back to their own country, Haitians added to the myth that AIDS could be found only among groups that either could not or would not conform to normal American values. Thus, AIDS was now a menace coming at society from those inside (homosexuals and drug users) as well as those outside the nation's borders (immigrants). The fact that Haitians were dark-skinned also gave AIDS a clear path to racial bigotry that had been missing when the disease was confined to homosexuals and drug users.

Because AIDS fit so neatly into the conservative agenda, it soon became a litmus test by which candidates for political office were judged. If one was not tough on AIDS, one was clearly in favor of homosexuality, drug use, and general immorality. Many candidates, sensing the political capital to be gained from AIDS, began to include in their standard stump speeches a statement that they favored mandatory testing, the reporting of those infected with AIDS, and the isolation and quarantining of all persons with AIDS, regardless of whether they posed a threat to society.

Much of the political fanfare over AIDS in the early years was sparked by sensational news reports. Wild claims were made of the number of persons with AIDS, the cost of AIDS-related care, the willingness of infected individuals to intentionally infect others, and the threat faced by those not otherwise at risk. Responsible data often went unreported by the media as being too technical and too filled with medical and scientific jargon to be readily understood by the public at large. Thus, a frenzy of misinformation (or no information) rapidly convinced the public that AIDS could be caught simply by shaking hands with, touching, hugging, sharing eating utensils with, or using the same bathroom as a person with AIDS. When scientists attempted to dispel such myths, they were routinely hooted down as being apologists for the homosexual community.

Although it is possible that nothing could have prevented the early politicization of AIDS, it is clear that the federal government's initial handling of the AIDS crisis aggravated the situation in diverse ways. Throughout his first term, Ronald Reagan refused to speak out on AIDS, believing that it would go away in the same manner as it had appeared.

A critical turning point came in 1985, when the actor Rock Hudson died of AIDS. Hudson had been a good friend of both Nancy and Ronald Reagan. His death gave a human dimension to AIDS and forced President Reagan to take note of the disease. No longer was AIDS a disease of inner-city homosexuals, drug addicts, and immigrants. Suddenly, AIDS was a problem that was capable of affecting the rich and famous. At about the same time, the battle of Ryan White gained national prominence.

White was an Indiana teenager and hemophiliac who had become HIV-infected from a blood transfusion. When his condition became known to school authorities, they refused to allow him to continue attending school. As a person who was neither gay nor a drug user, White reinforced the notion that AIDS was not confined to any specific segment of society. He later became a national hero due to his courage in dealing with the disease and its impact on him.

The realization that AIDS was not an isolated problem of certain fringe groups forced society to look at AIDS in a new light. Suddenly, it was acceptable to at least suggest that AIDS was simply a public health problem. The movement to a more tempered response to AIDS found its earliest expression in certain cities, such as Los Angeles and West Hollywood, that passed ordinances outlawing discrimination on the basis of a person having AIDS or being HIV-infected. Such ordinances, together with various court victories around the country, particularly in cases in which HIV-positive children won the right to remain or to be readmitted to school, helped to diminish the hysteria generated by AIDS.

The end of the early politicization of AIDS began in 1987 with the publication of Randy Shilts' groundbreaking book "And the Band Played On." A brilliant exposé of the federal government's mishandling of the crisis, the book prompted several critical changes. First, President Reagan finally began speaking about AIDS, stressing that the public should not panic over the disease. Second, under heavy pressure from Congress, Reagan appointed a thirteen member blue-ribbon panel, known as the Presidential Commission on the Human Immunodeficiency Virus Epidemic, to prepare a comprehensive report on what should be done about AIDS. Third, Congress, which had been slowly increasing the amount of research money available for AIDS, now began to do so with enthusiasm. Whereas just

$61 million had been earmarked for AIDS in 1984, by 1987 the figure was approaching $1 billion.

Thus, by 1988 a new tone was being set. First, the Presidential Commission issued its final report on the epidemic. The report savagely criticized the federal government's handling of AIDS during the first six years of the crisis and suggested, in rather blunt terms for such a document, that Reagan was largely at fault. The report also contained 579 recommendations for the future handling of the epidemic. Even Ronald Reagan began to take a softer stance towards AIDS. Although he had been against earlier efforts to obtain federal funds for AIDS, he now suddenly began urging Congress to approve more money for AIDS, and called for an appropriation of $1.3 billion. At the same time, he began boasting about how much money his administration was devoting to AIDS research.

During the presidential election of 1988, every candidate for the White House issued a statement on AIDS, including George Bush, the eventual victor. Nearly all of these statements sought to take a balanced and reasonable-sounding approach in keeping with the new national tone. AIDS also found a place at both the Democratic and Republican national conventions. The Democratic platform referred to AIDS as an unprecedented health emergency that required accelerated research, comprehensive education, confidential testing, and protection of the civil rights of persons with AIDS. The Republican platform lauded the Reagan administration for having spent over $5 billion on AIDS since 1983 and promised to continue the fight against AIDS. At the same time, it called for people with AIDS to remain in school or on the job as long as they were functionally capable of doing so.

2. More Recent Politicization

It would be a mistake to assume that AIDS suddenly stopped being used by conservatives in their battle to return the nation to a more chaste time. Many conservatives continue to see in AIDS not only legitimate reason for concern but an opportunity to win over members of the public. In a highly-publicized incident in 1989, for example, conservatives were able to force the National Endowment for the Arts (NEA) to modify its support of a New York City AIDS art show entitled "Witnesses: Against Our Vanishing," on the ground that the show was political rather than artistic in nature. Although the NEA eventually decided to fund the show, it did so only after the organizers of the show agreed to amend their grant proposal to request funding only for the show itself, rather than for the show and the show's catalogue. The catalogue had outraged conservatives because it contained unflattering references to the AIDS policies of numerous conservative leaders.

Nevertheless, for a variety of reasons, conservatives are finding it increasingly difficult to obtain the sort of political capital from AIDS that they once did.

First, persons with AIDS are increasingly being treated like individuals with other life-threatening illnesses. The intense rhetoric that once marked debates about AIDS has lessened. When Ryan White, the hemophiliac teenager who contracted AIDS from a blood transfusion, died in 1990, both President Bush and former President Reagan issued statements mourning his death and calling on Americans to fight the disease rather than those suffering from it. A short time earlier, in a speech on AIDS in Arlington, Virginia, President Bush had called for more AIDS research and appealed to the public to show compassion to persons with AIDS. Noting that both he and his wife Barbara had lost loved ones to AIDS, Bush railed against ignorance and prejudice about AIDS.

The view that people with AIDS should be treated as people has continued up to the present. In December 1995, for example, President Clinton denounced homophobia and other forms of bigotry committed against people with HIV and urged Americans not to "let our fears outweigh our common sense or compassion."

Second, it now is fashionable for politicians to openly support AIDS funding. In 1990, Congress voted overwhelmingly in favor of an AIDS-disaster bill, known as the Ryan White Comprehensive AIDS Resources Emergency (CARE) Act, that committed nearly $4 billion to AIDS research, treatment, education, and prevention over a five year period. Although certain long-time opponents of AIDS funding, such as Senator Jesse Helms, a Republican from North Carolina, and Representative William E. Dannemeyer, a Republican from California, fought hard to defeat the bill and introduced numerous amendments to water it down, their efforts proved futile.

Despite the federal government's recent fiscal woes, AIDS funding continues to be relatively generous. For 1995, Congress authorized $4.1 billion in AIDS monies. This amount represented a 6% increase over the previous year, although it was $300 million less than the number sought by President Clinton.

Third, the National Commission on AIDS, which replaced the Presidential HIV Epidemic Commission, continued the process of generating recommendations to be considered by national policymakers. Before ending its work in September 1993, the National Commission called for the appointment of a Cabinet-level AIDS coordinator to ensure that the federal response to AIDS would proceed in the most effective way possible. In response, President Clinton appointed Kristine M. Gebbie to be the nation's first "AIDS Czar." In August 1994, Gebbie was replaced by Patricia S. Fleming.

Since becoming the National AIDS Policy Coordinator, Fleming has overseen a restructuring of the White House's AIDS programs. Chief among these efforts was the creation in June 1995 of a thirty-member Presidential Advisory Council on HIV/AIDS. Chaired by Dr. R. Scott Hitt, a Los Angeles physician with extensive AIDS experience, the

Council is designed to advise the president on how the government can improve AIDS prevention, research, and treatment programs. In December 1995, President Clinton, at the Council's urging, held a one-day conference on AIDS at the White House.

Interestingly enough, these changes are taking place even as some persons with AIDS seek to increase the disease's politicization. In 1987, Larry Kramer, a New York City playwright, called for the establishment of a new group that would use its collective anger to achieve political results. Out of his suggestion grew an organization known as ACT–UP, or the AIDS Coalition to Unleash Power. ACT–UP insists that AIDS is a political problem as well as a health problem and that only through political action can people with AIDS make the system respond to their needs in a timely and meaningful fashion.

Since its founding, ACT–UP has staged numerous protests. These protests normally have been held in high profile places, such as churches, government offices, and scientific conventions. In 1990, for example, ACT–UP managed to keep Dr. Louis W. Sullivan, the Secretary of the United States Department of Health and Human Services (HHS), from speaking at the Sixth International Conference on AIDS in San Francisco by literally shouting him down. In response, Dr. Sullivan issued an order prohibiting employees of the Department from speaking with ACT–UP unless absolutely necessary.

While many people sympathize with ACT–UP's members, others have branded them "gangsters" and have charged that their activities will cause a backlash among the general public and provoke AIDS researchers to leave the field. During the Sixth International Conference, a counter-demonstration was held in which scientists and people with AIDS joined hands and marched through the streets of San Francisco to show solidarity and send the message that not all people with AIDS support tactics like the ones used by ACT–UP. Nevertheless, ACT–UP has managed to achieve a number of important victories. In particular, their actions have forced the FDA to speed up the approval of new AIDS drugs and allow the use of drugs that have not yet been approved.

The fear that a backlash may be developing to AIDS activists and the causes they espouse has at least some validity. In Concord, California, a quiet suburb of Oakland, voters in the 1989 general election handily repealed an ordinance that protected people with AIDS, as well as those suspected of having AIDS and those who associate with people with AIDS, from discrimination. Such ordinances exist in many cities. In voting against the ordinance, the vast majority of Concord residents indicated that although they were not in favor of discriminating against people with AIDS, they objected to the idea of singling out for preferred treatment a specific group of citizens.

In the future, AIDS will continue to be politicized by conservatives as well as by persons with AIDS.

But AIDS also will become a political matter for two more groups: people of color and women. As explained above, in the past few years AIDS has become a problem of growing importance for both people of color and women. At the same time, these two groups continue to make impressive (although belated) strides in the political arena, winning an increasing number of posts at all levels of government. Thus, as more people of color and women contract AIDS, and as more people of color and women gain political influence, AIDS will make yet another mark on the political landscape.

To an extent, the foregoing already can be observed. The Congressional Black Caucus, which for years privately supported increased AIDS spending, finally began making its position publicly known in 1990. At the same time, studies indicating that AIDS has become a leading cause of death among women (and is the leading cause among young African–American women in New York City) have forced many people, politicians included, to take a new look at AIDS.

The greatest potential for future politicization, however, stems from the fact AIDS has spawned a rebirth of tuberculosis (TB) cases. Unlike AIDS, which is difficult to contract and cannot be transmitted through casual contacts, TB is very contagious. Although the link between the surge in AIDS cases and the return of TB is still not completely understood, it is believed that TB finds in people with AIDS a natural host too weak to fight back. It is also theorized that as a person's ability to fight off disease is diminished by AIDS, any dormant TB cells gain a new opportunity to become active. If TB should again become a major health threat, there may come a time when there is a medically-justified need for the kind of isolation and quarantine measures that were demanded at the onset of the AIDS crisis. This, in turn, will undoubtedly bring forth a new wave of public hysteria of the sort about which irresponsible politicians may try to capitalize.

3. Consequences of Politicization

The politicization of AIDS is extremely troubling, regardless of the source of the politicization. There are at least three consequences of politicization, each of which is negative. First, politicization obscures the fact that AIDS is a public health problem and must be dealt with as such. Second, politicization tends to promote bigotry, prejudice, and ignorance by causing the public's attention to focus on the people involved in the issue rather than on the disease itself. Third, politicization distorts the normal research and treatment process by subjecting everyone involved to a heightened awareness that their acts are being scrutinized and will be judged by political rather than medical considerations.

It has taken a very long time for most politicians to realize that AIDS is a public health issue. Many members of the public still do not view (or are unwilling to accept) AIDS as a public health matter. This is unfortunate, because the best chance of defeating AIDS lies in following the traditional public health measures of education, prevention, and research. By converting AIDS into a political spectacle, public health officials are stymied in their efforts to develop and implement programs that are likely to reduce the spread of the disease while the medical and scientific communities work on developing a cure or a vaccine.

Politicizing AIDS also has the effect of changing the nature of the public dialogue surrounding the epidemic. Politicization tends to lead to personalization. When a condition is personalized, it takes on the characteristics of those with whom it is identified. Thus, the politicization of AIDS has caused the public to make a link between AIDS and homosexuals, drug users, and immigrants. This link has led to an image of AIDS in which the disease has the same qualities as those that are portrayed in the stereotypes that have been constructed about homosexuals, drug users, and immigrants.

By weighing the disease down with the characteristics of its victims, public discussion becomes less and less about AIDS and more and more about the individual and collective virtues of people with AIDS. Clearly, no disease, and especially not one as fatal and tragic as AIDS, should be used as proxy for passing judgment on its victims. This point was made expressly by President Bush during his Arlington address in 1990 when he reminded his audience that society does not blame people who are injured while driving without wearing seat belts. By the same token, society should not seek to blame

AIDS victims. Nevertheless, there is a tendency in this country to divide people with AIDS into the "innocents," such as Ryan White, who contracted AIDS through blood transfusions and other passive activities, and the "non-innocents," such as homosexuals and drug users, who are thought to bring AIDS on themselves by affirmatively engaging in high risk acts. Even if such a distinction can be made, it clearly has no relevance to the task of designing and implementing an effective public health strategy.

Finally, politicizing AIDS places unwarranted and unnecessary pressure on every health care professional dealing with AIDS. By suggesting, even if only obliquely, that the professional's conduct may at some time in the future be judged by political criteria, the message is sent that coping with the epidemic effectively is not as important as dealing with it in a politically correct manner. Professionals should not have to respond to such pressures. Moreover, by suggesting that political factors should be taken into account, an extra element of delay is added to the decision making process. Health policy ought to be made solely on the basis of the best available medical evidence, without fear that such policy may be politically second-guessed.

Even where politics works to the advantage of those with AIDS, such as by causing more money to be appropriated to AIDS research, there is a problem. By suggesting that AIDS is a suitable subject for the political arena, today's victories can become tomorrow's defeats. By choosing to seek a political solution, AIDS activists lose the right to complain when the political process hands them a defeat.

The politics over AIDS has been truly extraordinary. What other disease has been symbolized by a group comparable to ACT–UP, by a quilt acres in size representing its deceased victims, or by an ornament (the overused red ribbon) so politically correct that it has been widely worn by both ordinary people and the elite? How many diseases arrive at the point where they attain their own "awareness" postage stamps and their own first-run movies? It thus seems safe to predict that political gaming about AIDS will continue well into the future.

CHAPTER II

DISCRIMINATION LAW

A. INTRODUCTION

Discrimination against persons with AIDS may be redressed through a variety of federal, state and local laws, as well as constitutional provisions when the discriminating party is a public agency. This chapter focuses primarily on federal statutory law, which deals with AIDS as a "disability." Where appropriate, state or local laws and constitutional principles will be mentioned.

Early in the epidemic, most discrimination appeared to arise from fear of contagion or dislike of homosexuals or drug users, especially in the settings of health care facilities. As the public became more knowledgeable and hysteria about contagion moderated, other concerns emerged, although fear of contagion remains a significant factor. Some employers were frightened by the reputed high costs of treating AIDS that would affect their employee benefit plans, or were concerned that having an employee with a fatal illness would deter customers or clients or hurt employee morale. Landlords believed that renting to a person with AIDS, or to an AIDS service organization or treatment facility, would affect the value of their property.

Operators of places of public accommodation, such as restaurants, feared loss of patronage if persons with AIDS were customers. Ironically, health care institutions, where one would expect the most knowledge about HIV and AIDS transmission, remain a major source of discrimination, as evidenced by continuing litigation over refusal of treatment and the adoption of policies restricting the employment of HIV-infected health care workers.

1. Disability Discrimination Laws

Disability discrimination laws already existed when the AIDS epidemic began to produce discrimination claims in 1983. The Vocational Rehabilitation Act of 1973, 29 U.S.C.A. §§ 701–796, prohibited discrimination against qualified handicapped individuals by federal agencies, federal contractors, and programs that received federal funding (including, most notably, hospitals and schools). Some of the earliest AIDS discrimination cases against schools and hospitals were filed under § 504 (29 U.S.C.A. § 794) of this Act, which provides that "otherwise qualified" persons with disabilities may not be discriminated against by programs that receive federal funding.

The Rehabilitation Act defines the protected class as consisting of persons with physical or mental impairments that affect their ability to perform major life functions (among which "working" is included), persons with a record of such an impairment, and persons regarded by others as having such an impairment. The tripartite definition makes clear that the purpose of the prohibition on discrimination is to require employers to undertake rational decisionmaking in dealing with employees who either suffer impairments or are believed to suffer impairments; the last part of the definition supports the argument that persons without any actual impairment are protected from discrimination if the motivation for their disparate treatment stems from the employer's belief that they suffer from such an impairment.

In regulations implementing the Rehabilitation Act, federal agencies borrowed from Title VII of the Civil Rights Act of 1964 (42 U.S.C.A. §§ 2000e *et seq.*) the concept of "reasonable accommodation" contained in the provisions concerning discrimination on the basis of religion. This concept imposes an obligation on employers, federal contractors, and federal funding recipients to take steps to make it possible for persons with disabilities to participate in their programs (whether as employees or other participants), provided that the expense and inconvenience of providing such an accommodation does not impose an "undue hardship" on the business.

Many state and local civil rights laws included persons with handicapping conditions as a protected class, and extended to them protection from discrimination in employment, housing, public accommodations, credit, schools, and other government services. One of the first AIDS discrimination cases to be litigated involved the refusal by the board of directors of a cooperative apartment building in New York City to renew the office lease for a doctor who treated persons with AIDS. The case, which did not produce a published court opinion, was brought under the New York State Human Rights Law, and resulted in an injunction against the building.

Several years later, in a Massachusetts state case known as *Cronan v. New England Telephone & Telegraph Co.*, a state law against discrimination and a state privacy statute were successfully brought to bear in a discrimination case involving a telephone line repairman. The court held that AIDS was a handicap under the statute and that current knowledge about the disease indicated it was appropriate to order the employee's reinstatement and penalize the employer for disclosing information about his medical condition to other employees.

2. Application to AIDS

Taking advantage of this existing body of discrimination law, advocates for people with AIDS persuaded enforcement officials and courts to interpret the laws to protect their clients, rather than undertake the time-consuming and uncertain task of securing enactment of new laws specifically forbidding AIDS-based discrimination (although such laws were passed in a few cities, including Los Angeles, San Francisco, and Austin, Texas). The main obstacle was the lack of prior precedent or legislative history supporting the application of disability discrimination laws to contagious diseases. As a result, early charges of discrimination against hospitals, schools, and employers were treated as cases of first impression, resulting in long, drawn-out litigation before favorable decisions could be obtained in appellate courts.

By the late 1980s, appellate courts in several jurisdictions had concluded that people with AIDS (and perhaps those with HIV infection who had not been diagnosed with AIDS) could be protected by disability discrimination laws. A few jurisdictions also had enacted AIDS-specific discrimination laws at the urging of advocates who, dissatisfied with the slow pace of judicial decisionmaking, sought a specific basis to empower local enforcement agencies to vindicate discrimination claims.

3. The *Arline* Case

In 1987, the United States Supreme Court lent its support to the trend toward protection against discrimination for persons with contagious diseases. In *School Board of Nassau County v. Arline*, the Court held that persons disabled by contagious conditions were protected from employment discrimination by § 504 of the Rehabilitation Act if they were "otherwise qualified" to perform the work and did not present a "significant risk" of contagion in their workplace. The case involved a Florida school teacher who had suffered several relapses of the tuberculosis that she had contracted in childhood. After her third relapse, the school board ordered that she be permanently removed from the classroom. Because she was unable to obtain relief from the state's civil rights agency, she filed suit in federal court under § 504 of the Rehabilitation Act.

The trial judge dismissed her suit, reasoning that Congress had not intended to protect persons with contagious conditions from employment discrimination when it enacted § 504. On appeal, the Eleventh Circuit reversed. It concluded that the teacher's history of recurrent tuberculosis fit neatly within the definition of disability contained in the Act and ordered that a trial be held to determine whether the teacher was qualified to be in the classroom.

In an opinion by Justice William J. Brennan, Jr., the Supreme Court affirmed the court of appeals. Justice Brennan indicated that the Rehabilitation Act requires the government and private organizations that receive government money to make their decisions about persons with disabilities on the basis of the best scientific evidence, rather than on the basis of myths, fears, or stereotypes about disabled people or contagious conditions. Justice Brennan noted that fear of contagion had been a powerful engine for discriminatory exclusion in the past, but was an inappropriate basis for decisionmaking under the Rehabilitation Act. Rather, employers and others covered by the Act could only exclude those infected with a contagious agent if they presented a "significant risk" to others in the workplace, and the recommendations of public health officials were to be given heavy deference in making such a determination. Justice Brennan noted with approval the regulations requiring "reasonable accommodation" for persons with disabling conditions. On remand, a federal trial court determined that the teacher, whose tuberculosis was in remission, was "otherwise qualified" to resume teaching because the danger of transmission to children in her classroom was minimal.

In subsequent amendments to the Rehabilitation Act concerned primarily with clarifying the coverage of the Act to funding recipients, Congress included language intended to codify the approach to contagious diseases espoused by the Supreme Court in *Arline*. The new language stated that persons whose condition presented a "direct threat" to others would not be protected from exclusion, with "direct threat" to be evaluated along the lines suggested by the Supreme Court's decision.

4. The FHA and the ADA

By the end of the 1980s, a national consensus had formed with respect to the need for broadly applicable federal laws forbidding disability discrimination. By then, all but a handful of states forbade such discrimination, but state laws varied widely in their coverage, requirements, and remedies. The Bush Administration and leading organizations in the business community supported the concept of national legislation, in part to escape the difficulties that multistate activities and organizations experienced in trying to comply with more than forty state laws and scores of local ordinances.

A first step toward this goal was the 1988 amendment of the Fair Housing Act (FHA), 42 U.S.C.A. §§ 3601–3631, that protects against disability discrimination in the sale or rental of residential premises. In 1990, Congress passed the historic Americans with Disabilities Act (ADA), 42 U.S.C.A. §§ 12101–12213, which imposes non-discrimination requirements on all workplaces covered by Title VII, as well as places of public accommodation, public transportation and communications, and government services. At the same time, Congress retained the Rehabilitation Act, with suitable amendments to conform its terminology and remedies to the ADA.

The ADA, which is enforced by the Equal Employment Opportunity Commission (EEOC), includes provisions authorizing state and local governments to continue providing protection against disability discrimination; thus, federal law does not preempt local efforts that provide the same or stronger protection against discrimination. Because the ADA incorporates the enforcement provisions of Title VII, which emphasizes deferral to state and local enforcement agencies, such agencies will continue to play a significant role in dealing with AIDS-related discrimination. In the subsequently enacted Civil Rights Act of 1991, Congress strengthened the remedial arsenal of Title VII and the ADA by authorizing punitive damages for intentional discrimination, in addition to the already existing authorization of equitable remedies.

B. DISABILITY LAW

1. Definitions

Disability law is different from other types of discrimination law in several basic ways. Race discrimination laws protect all persons who suffer discrimination on the basis of their race or color, regardless of their specific race or color; sex discrimination laws, similarly, protect all persons who encounter discrimination on account of sex, whether they are male or female. By contrast, disability laws protect those who are suffering from "a physical or mental impairment that substantially limits one or more of the major life activities" of the person, or those who encounter discrimination because they have a record of such a disability or are regarded by others as having such a disability. 42 U.S.C.A. § 12102(2). Thus, the law protects persons who do not have a disability, if others treat them as if they do have one.

On the other hand, in order for the individual to be protected, the condition alleged to be a disability must "substantially limit" a "major life activity" of the individual. What this means in practice is that the question of whether an individual is within the class of persons protected by the law (*i.e.*, an individual with a "disability") may be the subject of intense litigation, due to disagreement about whether the alleged impairment is substantial enough to qualify. People with temporary disabilities or minor disabling conditions often find that they are not covered.

Almost a decade of test case litigation under the Rehabilitation Act and state and local laws created an impressive body of precedent holding that persons with AIDS are "individuals with disabilities" under these laws. By the time Congress came to consider the ADA, the concept was so well established that there was little question that AIDS would be covered by the new law, and there are frequent references in the legislative history so indicating.

AIDS is not mentioned in the ADA directly, but neither are any other disabling conditions. Rather, the statute describes in general terms the law's concept of a disability, and leaves to the processes of regulation and adjudication the determination whether particular conditions qualify. Regulations and interpretive guidelines adopted by the EEOC and early cases decided under the ADA confirm that HIV infection and AIDS are both covered.

Recent medical research findings support the EEOC's conclusions. Upon infection, HIV quickly incorporates itself into immune system cells and begins reproducing, destroying those cells in the process. Although the body generates new immune system cells, after several years of infection the rate of cell destruction begins to outpace the rate of cell regeneration, and ultimately the individual's cell count becomes so low that the body is disabled from combating opportunistic infections, whose occurrence (together with a low cell count) marks clinical AIDS. Thus, a person who is infected with HIV but who has not suffered opportunistic infections is nonetheless suffering from a physical impairment as the immune system is gradually compromised (contrary to the previous belief that HIV remains dormant and inactive until shortly before symptoms occur).

2. Qualifications

Disability discrimination law also differs from other civil rights laws by incorporating directly into the provisions prohibiting discrimination the concept of "qualifications." While every African–American is protected from discrimination based solely on race, not every person with a disability is protected from discrimination based solely on disability. A physical or mental impairment must be sufficiently severe so that it "substantially limits" a "major life activity" in order to be counted as a statutory disability. A temporary case of the flu does not count as a statutory disability. Neither does pregnancy, a time-limited physical disability that is dealt with separately under Title VII as an aspect of sex discrimination.

Smith v. Dovenmuehle Mortgage, Inc. illustrates the tension between the requirement of substantial impairment and continued ability to work. The employer claimed that a former employee with AIDS was estopped from suing under disability discrimination law because he had applied to the Social Security Administration for disability benefits. Rejecting this argument, the court explained that "the SSA's decision to award benefits is not synonymous with a determination that plaintiff is not a 'qualified individual' under the ADA, since these determinations were being made in different fora for different purposes."

However, in *McNemar v. The Disney Stores, Inc.*, a different district court held that an employee who filed an affidavit stating that he was permanently disabled as a result of AIDS in order to get disability benefits was judicially estopped from alleging the elements of a *prima facie* case under the ADA. Rejecting the *Smith* court's conclusion that use of estoppel in this context would put the recently terminated plaintiff in an "untenable" position, the *McNemar* court held that there was no indication in the ADA or its legislative history that Congress intended to allow duplicative benefits in the form of both an ADA remedy and disability benefits.

The prohibition against discrimination extends only to a "qualified individual with a disability." 42 U.S.C.A. § 12112(a). Such an individual, in the context of employment, is a person with a disability "who, with or without reasonable accommodation, can perform the essential function of the employment position that such individual holds or desires." 42 U.S.C.A. § 12111(8). Thus, in order to qualify for protection, a person must be significantly impaired, but not so impaired that he or she cannot perform essential job functions, at least with some reasonable degree of assistance or accommodation.

A person with a statutory disability who cannot perform the essential functions of a job (and is thus not qualified) may be excluded solely on the basis of that disability, provided that they receive the same sort of treatment from their employer that is normally accorded persons with disabling conditions. Put another way, an employer who treats people with HIV differently from people with other medical conditions, without some objective justification for the differential treatment, is in violation of the ADA.

3. Reasonable Accommodations

The incorporation of the "reasonable accommodation" concept is another way that disability law differs from more traditional civil rights laws. Employers and other business owners usually are not required by law to make special adjustments or accommodations to take account of differences of race or sex; they are required in a limited way to make accommodations for religious practice, but not, according to the Supreme Court, to incur more than *de minimis* expense or inconvenience in doing so. In the case of persons with disabilities, however, businesses are expected to incur expenses and even some inconvenience in providing accommodations to make it possible for persons with disabilities to work or enjoy the services offered by the business.

Congress' anticipation that planning and construction would be required to make businesses and government agencies accessible to employees, clients, and customers with disabilities caused it to delay the effective date of various ADA provisions, in some cases by as long as four years. By 1994, however, all requirements of the ADA were in effect for covered businesses and employers.

The degree of expense and inconvenience to be imposed on employers is limited by the concept of "undue hardship." 42 U.S.C.A. § 12111(10). A business is expected to incur "reasonable" expenses in order to accommodate persons with disabilities, and bears the burden of showing either that any effective accommodation would impose an undue hardship in light of the nature and scope of the business' operations, or that there is no accommodation that would make continued participation possible, in order to escape that obligation. Neither the ADA nor its implementing regulations contain a bright line test for determining whether a particular accommodation would present an undue hardship, although business spokespersons had requested such a test, based on a fraction of a business' revenues, both when the ADA was being considered by Congress and when the EEOC was considering comments on proposed regulations. Neither Congress nor the EEOC agreed to these requests, reasoning that the myriad of circumstances under which an accommodation might be needed was such that any attempt to adopt a "rule of thumb" would be futile. Thus, deciding whether an accommodation is reasonable is a case-by-case process.

The statute and implementing regulations suggest two kinds of accommodations: those that modify the physical workplace to take account of physical limitations (such as ramps and elevators), and

those that modify work rules or practices. As to
the latter, adjusted work schedules or job transfers
are possible accommodations.

4. Direct Threat Exception

Another way in which disability law is distinguished from other types of civil rights protection is
in its exclusion of protection for those persons
whose disabilities would present a "direct threat"
of harm to other employees, customers, or (according to some authorities) themselves. The "direct
threat" concept stems from the *Arline* decision, in
which the Supreme Court said that a person whose
contagious condition presents a "significant risk" to
others in the workplace would not be protected by
the Rehabilitation Act.

In response to *Arline*, Congress amended the Rehabilitation Act to exclude from protection anyone
whose condition presents a "direct threat" of harm.
Similar language was incorporated in the ADA, in
addition to special provisions requiring the HHS
Secretary to maintain a list of contagious conditions
transmitted by food-handling, and excluding persons suffering such conditions from employment in
food-handling occupations. Ironically, the so-called
"food-handling amendment" to the ADA was inspired by AIDS fears, despite the total lack of evidence that HIV is transmitted through food-handling. The Secretary has never listed HIV infection
under this provision, and the "direct threat" exception has had its greatest impact in the area of
employment of HIV-infected health care workers.

5. Rehabilitation Act Precedents Under the ADA

Because of the similarities between the ADA and the Rehabilitation Act, cases decided under the Rehabilitation Act are considered relevant precedents in interpreting the ADA. However, there are some significant differences, including Congress' decision not to preserve the Rehabilitation Act's limited scope of protection to those who suffer discrimination *solely* due to their handicapping condition; arguably, the ADA's employment provisions go beyond this and apply to "mixed-motive" cases (*i.e.*, cases where the employer may have been motivated by several considerations, only one of which is the employee's disability) and perhaps to disparate impact cases (*i.e.*, cases where an employee claims that a facially neutral rule has a disproportionately adverse impact on people with disabilities in general or people with a particular disability). Despite the foregoing differences, the EEOC and the courts will look to Rehabilitation Act precedents for guidance in determining whether a particular person has a disability within the meaning of the statute, as well as other interpretive issues that arise with respect to substantially similar statutory and regulatory provisions.

6. Other Important Features

In addition to prohibiting outright discrimination, the ADA protects the confidentiality rights of persons with disabilities by limiting the use of medical examinations to circumstances where they are necessary to determine job qualifications and requiring that the results of such examinations be kept strictly confidential. Furthermore, particular individuals cannot be discriminatorily singled out for medical examinations. Rather, such requirements must be uniformly applied to all applicants or employees. The ADA also has provisions that deal with employer-provided health benefits.

C. PUBLIC ACCOMMODATIONS

1. General Definitions

A public accommodation normally is defined as any privately-owned business that provides goods or services to the general public. Retail stores, personal service providers, hotels, restaurants, theaters, hospitals, and health clinics are all examples of public accommodations. In some states, insurance companies and schools may also be considered public accommodations, although they are frequently dealt with under specialized statutes rather than general public accommodations law.

In addition to businesses, government agencies or institutions that provide goods or services to the general public may be covered by such laws; if not, they are subject to a variety of special provisions forbidding discrimination in government services, as well as constitutional requirements to observe the commands of due process and equal protection of the laws. Public schools are a prime example of institutions required by disability laws to refrain from discriminating against qualified individuals with disabilities while bearing in mind constitutional protections for all their students and employees.

All government operations are bound by constitutional obligations of due process (including respect for personal privacy) and equal protection that may place a significant burden of justification on a public sector operation when it seeks to discriminate on some categorical basis.

2. Public Schools

AIDS has posed significant public accommodations issues in a variety of settings. Some of the earliest cases involved public schools seeking to exclude HIV-infected children, usually due to a fear that such children would infect others in incidents involving biting or bleeding. When the FDA licensed a screening test for HIV antibodies in 1985 and it became possible to determine whether a person was infected with the virus, school systems throughout the nation debated how to deal with the issue of HIV-infected children. Court battles raged in several states, but the most notable were in Indiana, where Ryan White, a hemophiliac youngster, won the right to attend public school; in Florida, where the young Ray brothers, also hemophiliacs, prevailed in court although their home was firebombed and they had to move to a different city to attend school in peace; and in New York City, where a local community school board brought a declaratory judgment action seeking a determination that the central board of education erred in deciding to admit HIV-infected children without revealing their identity to local school officials.

The New York City controversy produced one of the first published court decisions dealing with the status of HIV infection and AIDS under disability discrimination laws and constitutional principles. The court in *District 27 Community School Board v. Board of Education* upheld the central board's policy. It relied on a prior decision by the Second Circuit, *New York State Ass'n for Retarded Children, Inc. v. Carey*, which held that the Rehabilitation Act, the equal protection clause of the federal constitution, and laws governing the education rights of handicapped children, could be applied to prohibit public schools from segregating retarded children infected with hepatitis B from retarded children not so infected in the context of special education classes.

Noting that hepatitis B is much more contagious than HIV, and that HIV infection is very similar to hepatitis B infection, involving as it does a latent infection by a blood-borne virus that may not produce visible symptoms, the court in *District 27* held that HIV-infected children were protected by the Rehabilitation Act and the constitution. It also noted that the central board's policy did not mandate HIV testing for students, so the issue of excluding or identifying HIV-infected children would only arise if a child's HIV status was adventitiously known to school authorities or the child developed symptoms suggestive of AIDS.

Thus, at any time there were likely to be many children in the school system whose HIV status was not known to teachers or administrators. It would serve no useful purpose to alert teachers and administrators to the identity of those whose HIV status had been determined; special precautions in dealing with blood would always be appropriate because any child might be HIV-infected. The court concluded that the central school board's policy was rational and consistent with non-discrimination law, and dismissed the local board's complaint.

A short time later, the New Jersey Supreme Court adopted substantially the same analysis in reviewing that state's policy on public school attendance by children with HIV-infection. *Board of Education of the City of Plainfield v. Cooperman.* In a subsequent decision, a federal district court in California found that the likelihood of HIV transmission through biting was so slight that an HIV-infected child who had bitten another student in response to provocative teasing should be allowed to continue to attend school. The court reasoned that exclusion would only be justified, consistent with disability law principles, if biting were shown to be a significant means of transmission, which it was not. *Thomas v. Atascadero Unified School District.*

3. Other Public Accommodations

Apart from schools, most of the litigation about discrimination in places of public accommodation has focused on health care institutions and related businesses, such as dental offices, nursing homes, and funeral homes.

Prior to the passage of the ADA, there was some doubt whether private dental offices, which were unlikely to be covered by § 504 of the Rehabilitation Act, were affected by a non-discrimination requirement, because some state and local laws were unclear on this point. In New York, the lower state courts were divided about whether private dental offices were covered by the state and New York City public accommodations provisions. However, this point became moot as the ADA came into effect, because such offices are clearly covered under the federal law. The issue of what constitutes discrimination in such settings is still to be finally determined.

In a New York case, the court held that a dentist had not engaged in discrimination when he took extraordinary measures, including swathing the entire treatment area in protective paper coverings, when treating a patient with HIV-infection. The court emphasized that the dentist had not refused treatment, and found that the protective measures were within the discretion of the dentist. *Syracuse Community Health Center v. Wendi A.M.*

In a federal case in Louisiana, the court rejected a dentist's claim that he was privileged to refer patients with HIV to an "AIDS specialist" or an "AIDS clinic," finding that the professional standard of care for dentists encompassed the requirement of obtaining expertise necessary for safe treatment of patients with HIV infection. *United States v. Morvant*. The *Morvant* decision was the first to deal with dental offices under the ADA and among the first to hold that HIV infection constitutes a disability under the statute.

New York state courts have dealt with several cases involving nursing homes and funeral parlors. The courts have held that AIDS does not present extraordinary circumstances justifying exclusion or special restrictions in the context of nursing homes, *Marcus Garvey Nursing Home, Inc. v. New York State Div. of Human Rights*, or excusing refusals of service by funeral homes. In the latter case, although the person with AIDS had died, it was found that the funeral home's refusal of services to the surviving family members came within the public accommodations statute. *Dimicelli & Sons Funeral Home v. N.Y.C. Comm'n on Human Rights*. In *Doe v. Price*, a Philadelphia court awarded damages against a funeral director who used an empty casket at a funeral due to a fear of HIV.

Perhaps the most famous litigated public accommodations case involved a nail parlor in West Hollywood, California, that refused to give a manicure to a person with AIDS. The court found that the refusal was not justified by the risk of transmission of HIV, and that although a manicure was not an essential health service, persons with disabilities were entitled to equal treatment in all services provided to the public, not just essential services. *Jasperson v. Jessica's Nail Clinic*.

Most public accommodation litigation, however, has involved hospitals and clinics, where refusals of treatment or unequal treatment may have the most important consequences. Perhaps the most significant decision in this area is *Howe v. Hull*, one of the first public accommodations cases to be decided under the ADA. A person with AIDS was travelling through rural Ohio when he developed an allergic reaction to some medication. His travelling companion took him to a rural hospital and, thinking to alert the emergency room staff to the need for special precautions, revealed that the patient had AIDS. The doctor on call, claiming to believe that the hospital was not equipped to provide AIDS treatment, refused to admit the patient and referred him to another, larger hospital. The patient had not sought admittance for treatment for AIDS, but only for the allergic reaction to his medication. The court held that the physician's refusal to admit the patient was motivated by the patient's HIV status in violation of both the ADA and the Rehabilitation Act, as well as the Emergency Transfer and Active Labor Act, a federal law that prohibits hospitals from transferring patients under emergency circumstances when the patient's condition has not been stabilized prior to the transfer.

The underlying principle uniting all of these public accommodations cases is that a business or government operation that holds itself out to the public as providing services may not refuse to provide such services on account of the HIV or AIDS status of the individual seeking services or those associated with them unless the significant risk threshold has been crossed.

D. EMPLOYMENT

Most of the discrimination litigation involving AIDS has arisen in the workplace context. Such litigation inspired one of the first major motion pictures to deal with the AIDS epidemic, "Philadelphia," whose plot resembled in some particulars two of the significant early AIDS employment discrimination cases, *Bowers v. Baker & McKenzie* and *Cain v. Hyatt*. In both of these cases, lawyers alleged that they were fired because of their AIDS condition, while their employers asserted that the discharges were due to problems with their work. In both cases, the relevant tribunals decided that the employers' defenses were pretextual and awarded significant damages to the plaintiffs. In *Bowers*, the damages were awarded to the plaintiff's estate, as the litigation dragged on for so many years that he died long before the final disposition by a New York state administrative agency.

In an ironic case of real life imitating Hollywood, a new employment discrimination claim by a Philadelphia lawyer with AIDS surfaced late in 1993, just as "Philadelphia" was about to open in movie theaters. The facts of the case as alleged by the plaintiff (and strenuously denied by the defendants) were eerily similar to the plot of the film, which had been conceived years before. The case was settled prior to a final determination on the merits. *Doe v. Kohn Nast & Graf, P.C.*

1. Non–Health Care Employment

The most disputed issues in non-health care employment discrimination cases early in the epidemic concerned primarily risks of HIV transmission to co-workers or customers, and the employer's fears of liability for risk of injury to the employee with AIDS. As public education about AIDS reduced transmission fears somewhat, new concerns emerged, including employer fears of medical expenses and co-worker reactions.

The latter concern seemed vindicated by one of the earliest employment discrimination cases, *Cronan v. New England Telephone & Telegraph Co.*, when co-workers of a telephone lineman with AIDS refused to report for work after a state court found that the employer violated state disability and confidentiality laws by excluding the employee from his regular work assignment and ordered his reinstatement. However, fast intervention by state public health officials to meet with the affected employees and reassure them about the lack of danger of HIV transmission eventually led to a satisfactory resolution of the problem.

A decision of particular importance because of its thorough analysis of the issue of risk of transmission in a typical workplace setting is *Benjamin R. v. Orkin Exterminating Co.* Concurring in the court's decision that an employee with HIV infection was covered by the state's disability discrimination law,

Chief Justice Neely wrote a lengthy analysis of the issue of risk, both in the context of HIV and, more generally, comparing the possibilities of HIV transmission to other common risks of everyday life. He concluded that those risks were well within the tolerable range for a typical workplace.

Discharged employees with HIV infection have been less successful in combating unjustified discrimination in the food service industry. Chief Justice Neely suggested that the problem in a restaurant would not be with the actual risk of HIV transmission, but rather with the public perception of danger that might destroy the economic viability of the business. Although such customer perceptions have generally not been accorded legal significance as a defense to a discrimination charge in race or sex cases, some courts have apparently allowed them to weigh heavily in AIDS discrimination cases.

In *Wolfe v. Tidewater Pizza*, for example, the Virginia Supreme Court refused to review a lower court's decision rejecting a discrimination claim brought by a person with AIDS who had been discharged by a pizzeria. Similarly, in *Burgess v. Your House of Raleigh, Inc.*, the North Carolina Supreme Court dismissed a claim by an HIV-infected restaurant worker. It held that HIV infection without symptoms of AIDS was not covered as a disability under state law and noted that the state legislature had opted not to provide protection for persons with contagious diseases in food-handling jobs. However, in New York, an appellate court found that a restaurant had violated disability discrimination law by discharging a waiter with AIDS. *Club Swamp Annex v. White*.

As noted above, the ADA includes a provision dealing with food-handling employment that requires the HHS Secretary to maintain a list of contagious conditions that disqualify individuals from working in food-handling occupations. The Secretary has not designated HIV or AIDS as appropriate for that list, having concluded that these conditions do not present a "direct threat" of transmission to consumers.

The problem of "reasonable accommodation" in a non-health care setting will likely focus on work schedules and transfers. In *Buckingham v. United States*, a Rehabilitation Act case, a postal clerk with AIDS requested a transfer from Columbus, Mississippi, to Los Angeles, California, in order to take advantage of superior medical treatment possibilities in the later location. The Postal Service denied his request, relying on collective bargaining provisions governing transfer eligibility. The court found that the duty of reasonable accommodation is an affirmative one, and that "an employer is obligated not to interfere, either through action or inaction, with a handicapped employee's efforts to pursue a normal life," even where this means that the employer may have to "alter existing policies or procedures that they would not change for non-handicapped employees." The court emphasized that in this case, involving a nationwide employer with large numbers of fungible job positions for which the plaintiff was qualified, the request for transfer was obviously reasonable.

2. Health Care Employment

Health care employment of persons with AIDS presents special problems for the courts. During the course of the AIDS epidemic, hundreds of HIV-infected health care workers have provided care to patients in a variety of settings, from invasive surgical procedures to nursing care, but to date there has only been one incident where it is believed that an HIV-infected health care worker transmitted the virus to patients while rendering treatment.

That case concerns an HIV-infected dentist, six of whose patients were found to be infected with the same strain of the virus. The Centers for Disease Control and Prevention (CDC) have suggested various ways the transmission might have occurred in that case, but the agency is unable to say with certainty how it occurred, or even whether the dentist was necessarily the source of the patients' infections. However, publicity generated by the incident, magnified by the aggressive lobbying activity of Kimberly Bergalis, one of the infected patients, led to the promulgation of politically-inspired guidelines by the CDC that provided a basis for health care institutions to seek to restrict the patient care activities of HIV-infected health care workers who performed "invasive procedures" on patients. Leading medical societies, which had at first supported the CDC's regulations, subsequently balked at participating in designating which procedures should be placed on the "invasive" list when many of their members protested the regulation as being unscientific.

Repeated studies of the patients of HIV-infected health care workers have failed to yield confirmed cases of transmission during surgery or rendition of normal or emergency health care in hospitals, clinics, or doctors' offices. However, the CDC, using the more highly contagious hepatitis B virus as a model, and calculating backwards from statistics of health care workers becoming HIV-infected in needle-stick accidents with contaminated hypodermic works, published a report in 1991 calculating the likelihood that an HIV-infected health care worker might transmit HIV to a patient while performing invasive medical procedures as between 1/42,000 and 1/417,000, depending on the nature of the potential contact.

In cases where HIV-infected health care workers have been prevented from continuing their occupations due to fears of transmission to patients, the federal courts have uniformly adopted a "zero risk" approach, basing their analysis on the Supreme Court's discussion of contagious conditions in *Arline*. In *Arline*, the Court held that risk of harm to others must be "significant" to justify the exclusion of a contagious person from a workplace. The Court instructed lower federal courts to evaluate the significance of risk by taking into account four factors: 1) the nature of the risk (how the disease is transmitted), 2) the duration of the risk (how long the carrier is infectious), 3) the severity of the risk (the potential harm if transmission occurs), and, 4) the probability that the disease will be transmitted. The Court also indicated that in making these determinations judges should defer to the expert opinion of public health authorities.

The "zero risk" approach adopted by the lower federal courts focuses on the fourth element of the *Arline* analysis, assuming that elements 1–3 all weigh heavily against allowing the infected health care worker to continue performing invasive procedures. The lack of documented cases of HIV transmission militates against the conclusion that the first element should weigh against the plaintiff, because there is as yet no direct evidence that HIV is normally transmitted in such settings. As to the fourth element, the CDC's 1991 calculations remain hypothetical and speculative, and seem even less reflective of reality now, in light of subsequent studies that have failed to find any confirmed cases of transmission to patients during invasive procedures.

However, the courts have not embraced this reasoning. In *Leckelt v. Board of Commissioners*, a case of a gay male licensed practical nurse whose roommate had died from AIDS and who was discharged when he refused to obtain and reveal to his employer the results of an HIV test, the court found the hospital's actions to be lawful under both the Rehabilitation Act and state disability law. While the court agreed that a person with HIV is covered by § 504 of the Rehabilitation Act, the court ruled that Leckelt was discharged for insubordination, not for his actual or imagined HIV status, and that the hospital was justified in seeking to know his status in order to administer its "infection control policy."

Looking to the *Arline* factors, the court held that the hospital was justified, in terms of its responsibility to protect patients from infection, in seeking to know the HIV status of any employee who performed "invasive procedures" as to whom the hospital suspected HIV exposure, even though the hospital never spelled out what steps it might take with respect to Leckelt were it to learn that he tested positive.

In *Doe v. University of Maryland Medical System Corp.*, a case involving a neurosurgery resident who apparently contracted HIV through workplace exposure to a patient's blood, the court upheld the decision of hospital administrators to forbid the plaintiff from performing any invasive procedures, even though a board of medical experts convened by the hospital had recommended barring him from only one particular procedure that they deemed especially exposure-prone. The court accepted the hospital's argument that as long as there was any "ascertainable risk" of HIV transmission through performance of invasive procedures, the "significant risk" standard of *Arline* and the ADA was satisfied, primarily because should actual transmission take place the result would be to subject the patient to an incurable and fatal condition.

Just days after the *Doe v. University of Maryland* decision was announced, the CDC released a new study summarizing the results of investigations of more than 22,000 patients of 64 physicians, dentists, technicians, podiatrists, and other health care workers infected with HIV. Apart from the case of the Florida dentist discussed above, no other cases of HIV transmission from health care worker-to-patient had been found. Proponents of restrictions on HIV-infected health care workers pointed out, however, that these findings did not disprove the CDC's risk calculations, arguing that a much larger sample of patients would be necessary to test the validity of a prediction of risk in the $\frac{1}{42},000$ or less range.

Cases decided under the Rehabilitation Act and the ADA have involved surgeons, surgical technicians, and a licensed practical nurse. In all of these cases, the courts found that the hypothetical risk of transmission during invasive procedures (broadly defined to include such actions as a nurse starting an intravenous line or a surgical technician using medical instruments to hold open an incision while a surgeon operated) was legally "significant." The Supreme Court has not considered this issue yet, but the results in the lower federal courts seem inconsistent with Justice Brennan's statement in *Arline* that decisions to exclude persons with contagious conditions from their jobs should be based on the best available scientific information, and not on fears or stereotypes. Medical patients face higher risk of injury traveling to the place where they are to receive treatment than they face from receiving treatment from an HIV-infected health care worker. At present, however, there is no unanimity among legal commentators on how the balance should be struck with respect to health care workers, and the cases decided to date back the decisions of administrators to forbid such workers to perform invasive procedures, at least without the knowing consent of their patients.

Just recently, however, the Ninth Circuit, in a potentially landmark case, adhered to the principles laid out in *Arline*. In *Doe v. Attorney General*, the court revived a suit by the estate of a deceased physician against the FBI. The FBI had terminated the doctor's contract to perform physical examinations on its agents because they suspected that he had AIDS (the doctor would neither confirm nor deny his AIDS status). As the first appellate case to hold that HIV-infected health care workers who are dismissed from their jobs can sue under the ADA and the Rehabilitation Act, the decision may signal the start of an important new trend.

3. Workplace Health and Safety

Although it is not, strictly speaking, a discrimination issue, it is appropriate to mention briefly the efforts by government regulators, labor organizations, and employee advocates to secure safe working conditions relative to the AIDS epidemic. Awareness about the dangers of blood-borne transmission has produced significant changes in many American workplaces.

In particular, many employees now routinely receive special training on dealing with blood spill incidents and are supplied with rubber gloves and other materials for clean-up in such circumstances. Regulations issued by the Occupational Safety and Health Administration (OSHA) now require stringent planning by health care employers for dealing with contagious agents (*e.g.*, HIV, hepatitis B, and tuberculosis) in their workplaces. Tuberculosis is a particular concern among workers with suppressed immune systems due to HIV infection. Training, special safety equipment, and adoption of appropriate procedures for dealing with incidents are now all mandated by regulation. Perhaps the most controversial, and expensive, part of the regulation requires employers in health care institutions to provide hepatitis B vaccinations to employees at the employer's expense.

By the time OSHA promulgated these regulations in 1991 under its authority to prescribe rules and standards for workplace safety, most of the health care industry was already complying with many of the requirements, which had been issued in the form of recommendations by the CDC. However, some organizations in the health care industry disagreed with the mandatory nature of some of the regulations and challenged OSHA's authority to adopt them. In *American Dental Ass'n v. Martin*, the court found that the regulations were on the whole justified, although it agreed that in certain instances they went too far in placing responsibility on employers for conditions their employees might encounter at worksites beyond the employers' control. In those instances, the court required that the regulations be cut back slightly. The main requirements, however, were upheld.

E. HOUSING

At the federal level, the Fair Housing Act, amended in 1988 to prohibit discrimination on the basis of disability, now provides a major source of protection for people with AIDS. At the state and local levels, the disability discrimination provisions of civil rights laws usually apply to housing issues as well. There are two basic contexts in which problems arise: individual residential housing facilities and group housing (such as hospices and other AIDS residences).

In the former situation, the application of the law is rather straightforward, once it is established that a person with HIV or AIDS is a disabled person within the meaning of the relevant law. For example, in *Poff v. Caro*, a landlord rescinded an offer to rent a large apartment to three single men because the landlord feared that they were gay and might get AIDS. The state Division of Civil Rights sought an injunction against the landlord upon the complaint of the prospective tenants. The court found that the ban on handicap discrimination under the state's Law Against Discrimination applied because the landlord was discriminating based on a perception that the prospective tenants were at risk for a handicapping condition, and noted Justice Brennan's comment in *Arline* that "public fear and misapprehension about contagiousness" must not be held to justify excluding qualified persons from rental housing. The court went on to say: "To refuse to extend that protection to homosexuals because they may be more susceptible to a dread disease would mark a return to a past of judging individuals on the basis of ignorance and prejudice."

In the group home situation, the problem most frequently litigated has been the refusal of local government units to permit the construction or operation of such housing, usually through manipulation of a zoning or permit process for group residences. While zoning issues are a matter of local concern and authority, the Supreme Court ruled in *City of Cleburne v. Cleburne Living Center* that the use of zoning and permit rules to discriminate against group homes for certain feared groups (in that case the mentally retarded) violated equal protection requirements. Thus, litigation about group housing for persons with AIDS tends to focus on the motivations of those who apply the zoning rules in a discriminatory manner. In a series of cases, federal district courts have found either constitutional or statutory violations where it was shown that particular zoning rules had been adopted primarily to prevent the location of an AIDS residence in a particular community, or that permits for construction or operation had been denied in a discriminatory manner. These cases tend to focus more on disputes about facts and motivations than about how the substantive law should be applied, with preliminary skirmishing about jurisdiction frequently consuming most of the litigators' efforts.

F. LIMITS OF DISCRIMINATION LAW

In the first fifteen years of the AIDS epidemic, courts, legislators, and administrators have constructed an elaborate edifice of laws, regulations, and rules intended to redress discrimination against persons with AIDS. However, as individual cases repeatedly demonstrate, there are limits to what the law can accomplish. Because civil rights law is remedial rather than punitive, the effect of the law in specific cases is to provide compensation or other relief after the fact for painful discrimination, rather than to have prevented such discrimination from occurring in the first place.

On the other hand, it appears that many employers are establishing policies designed to comply with the law, and are instructing their managers and supervisors to conform their actions to such policies. Thus, the law may be having a salutary effect in preventing some discrimination. In this sense, the law fulfills its traditional role as the great teacher of human conduct, attempting to embody the lessons of considered judgment that employers, landlords, and other business operators should use in deciding how to deal with persons with disabilities.

CHAPTER III

FAMILY AND ESTATE PLANNING LAW

A. INTRODUCTION

AIDS has touched virtually every aspect of family law. As a disease that is transmitted through sexual relations, AIDS has had a major impact on such important questions as whether couples get married, have children, and stay together. At the same time, AIDS has fundamentally altered the options available for both heterosexual and gay individuals who wish to engage in relationships outside the traditional one of marriage.

In addition to these matters, AIDS has affected probate and estate planning law. The epidemic has again brought home both the importance of careful estate planning and the reality that even the most detailed post-death plans are subject to judicial challenge and disruption.

B. COUPLES

1. The Effect of AIDS on Relationships

Before AIDS was first identified in the early 1980s, the traditional family unit, centered around the institution of marriage, had suffered a substantial decline. Sexual awareness and freedom were at an all-time peak. More people were remaining unmarried. Far more families were composed of a single parent with one or more small children. The divorce rate was high. There were far more nontraditional relationships, such as heterosexual and gay couples cohabiting outside the sanctity of marriage.

The publicity given to AIDS has produced notable side-effects for the family. Although some people may be opting for sexual abstinence, AIDS more often has contributed to people remaining together in already existing relationships or coming together to form monogamous sexual unions. This trend has been seen especially in the gay community, although certainly a large proportion of the heterosexual population has felt the same pressure. Since one of the two most important routes of transmission of AIDS is through sexual intercourse, many people are being more cautious about both their sexual practices and their partners.

In the decade prior to the discovery of AIDS, the law had begun for the first time to seriously confront issues involving non-traditional family arrangements, particularly cohabitation by heterosexual and gay couples. Today, the common law in almost all jurisdictions recognizes and enforces agreements between unmarried cohabitants. These so-called "palimony" agreements received their most important judicial approval in *Marvin v. Marvin*. In that case, the California Supreme Court held that unmarried individuals can recover from persons with whom they have cohabited in accordance with the contract between them. The court further held that even if there is no express agreement, a party can still recover if an implied contract is found to exist or equitable considerations, including the doctrine of *quantum meruit*, make such a recovery just under the circumstances.

In the context of the AIDS epidemic, the palimony cases hold out the possibility of a number of potentially crucial rights to unmarried couples. For instance, the members of the couple can inherit from one another with less risk that a successful will challenge may be launched by other members of the blood family (especially where state law permits a will to be invalidated if the testator was mentally incapacitated by AIDS or was subject to the undue influence of the lover-legatee). Lovers whose relationships are recognized can more easily obtain coverage under the health insurance policies of one another. In case of illness, the healthy lover will have greater hospital visitation and medical decisionmaking privileges in regard to the ill lover. The surviving lover will be able to more readily participate in such matters as the making of funeral arrangements and the drafting of obituaries.

Some couples, not satisfied with the possibility that their agreements will be upheld under palimony law, have sought to gain greater legal recognition of their relationships. In particular, they have sought to have their relationships determined to be legal families. In *Baehr v. Lewin*, for example, same-sex couples in Hawaii sought to obtain marriage licenses but were refused by the local clerk's office. A sharply divided state supreme court held that the practice of denying the right to marry to same-sex couples presumptively violated the Hawaii Constitution and remanded the case for a trial.

Similarly, in *Braschi v. Stahl Associates Co.*, the lover whose name appeared on the lease of an apartment died from complications of AIDS. The other lover, who had resided with the decedent in the apartment for more than ten years, asserted a right to continue possession of the premises. Under the law, any member of the "family" who had resided in a rent-control apartment was entitled to remain in the apartment following the death of the leaseholder. In a closely divided opinion, the New York State Court of Appeals concluded that gay lovers can constitute a family. In arriving at its decision, the court indicated that the following factors should be considered in determining whether unmarried cohabitants (either gay or heterosexual) are a family for the purposes of the state's rent control statute: 1) the longevity and exclusively of the relationship, 2) the level of emotional and financial commitment of the couple to one another, 3) the way in which the members of the couple have conducted their lives and held themselves out to the rest of the world, and, 4) the reliance on one another for ordinary daily family services.

Whether any other jurisdiction will follow the lead of these cases in extending formal legal recognition to nontraditional couples is uncertain. The next test of this kind may come when a same-sex couple asserts the rights and privileges of a married couple under international comity rules. Sweden, Finland, and Denmark, for example, now have statutory provisions giving legal recognition to same-sex couples. These laws confer nearly the equivalent of a marriage upon such couples. There will undoubtedly come a time when a couple that has "married" under such a law will take up domicile in this country. Whether any state will give legal recognition to such a marriage is an open question that will require the courts to weigh numerous public policy concerns.

In addition to seeking direct recognition of their relationships, some lovers have sought to become members of a family through adult adoption. Most adoption statutes permit an adult to adopt another adult and there often is no requirement that the older party adopt the younger party. In many states, however, an adoption request will be denied if a sexual relationship exists between the parties.

In *Matter of Adoption of Robert Paul P.*, for example, two gay lovers admitted that they had been sexually intimate for many years and wished to legitimize their relationship. In ruling on their application, the New York State Court of Appeals held that adoption should mirror nature and that a parent-child relationship should be the result. Given this thesis, the court's majority had no trouble concluding that a union between gay lovers is abhorrent to the natural relationship of a parent and a child. The dissenters emphasized that laws permitting adult adoption involve no requirement that a natural parent-child relationship be established, especially in light of the fact that the statute did not require the older person to adopt the younger individual. In *In re Adoption of Swanson*, there was no express evidence that two men, who had been companions for 17 years, were involved in a sexual relationship. As such, the Delaware Supreme Court allowed one of the men to adopt the other.

Even if a gay or heterosexual lover is permitted to adopt his or her lover in order to formalize a "family" unit, there are some serious drawbacks that should be considered before couples embark upon such a route. It is not as easy to undo an adoption as it is to undo a marriage or cohabitation arrangement. Although one can divorce a spouse or separate from a cohabiting lover, one cannot so readily dissolve a parent-child relationship created by an adoption. Even if, as a practical matter, the members of the adoptive family go their separate ways, important legal ties resulting from the parent-child relationship, such as the right to inherit property, remain in place. Moreover, there are important legal, ethical, and moral concerns about a parent and a child having a sexual relationship. All states have laws against incest and it is quite possible that a state would declare sexual relations between adopting adults to be illegal, despite the consensual nature of the relationship.

2. Duty of Sexual Partners to Disclose Their AIDS Status

Regardless of whether people are married, living together, or simply involved in some form of sexual relationship, the AIDS epidemic has renewed the debate over whether a person has a legal duty to disclose his or her infectious condition to sexual partners.

As a result of this question, many states have considered the idea of requiring HIV blood testing as a prerequisite to the issuance of marriage licenses. Only Illinois and Louisiana, however, have ever adopted and enforced such laws, and both did so for only brief periods of time.

The Illinois and Louisiana statutes required applicants for a marriage license to submit to HIV testing. If either party tested positive, both individuals had to be informed of the results. The two laws allowed a marriage license to be issued even if one of the parties tested positive for HIV. In contrast, Utah adopted a statute, which was later struck down by a federal court, that prohibited anyone with AIDS from marrying. *T.E.P. v. Leavitt*.

In time, Illinois and Louisiana repealed their laws due to the inconvenience and expense of administrating them. It also was found that applicants for marriage licenses often did not wish to submit to HIV testing for fear that the confidentiality of the test or its results might be breached. As a result, many people in Illinois and Louisiana chose to live together, avoided entering into relationships, or crossed state lines and obtained marriage licenses in neighboring jurisdictions that did not require HIV testing.

Under the common law, it is well settled that an individual owes a duty of reasonable care to avoid contact with others if the individual is afflicted with an infectious disease that can be transmitted by such contact. Alternatively, the individual owes a duty to warn others before engaging in contact that involves the risk of transmission of the infectious condition. This has been the position of the law since the earliest days, as illustrated by cases involving the plague, smallpox, and other contagious diseases, and by later cases dealing with sexually transmitted diseases, such as herpes.

The same legal duties arise in the context of AIDS. Because AIDS is both incurable and deadly, individuals with AIDS have a legal duty to either avoid sexual activities with others that might risk the transmission of HIV or engage in such contact only after first warning sexual partners of their HIV condition and obtaining consent.

The common law defenses of assumption of risk and contributory negligence will not bar recovery by a plaintiff seeking damages from a defendant for sexual transmission of AIDS. Although there is a tendency to believe that a plaintiff has assumed the risk of, or contributed to, the occurrence of the injury by freely engaging in sexual intercourse with a party who has AIDS, the law takes the view that a person who engages in sexual intercourse consents to the sex but not to the transmission of an infectious disease.

Although the defenses of assumption of risk and contributory negligence will not serve as an absolute bar to a cause of action for transmission of AIDS, the plaintiff's recovery may be reduced as the result of the doctrine of comparative negligence. Thus, the facts that the plaintiff freely participated in sex and should have been aware of some risk of transmission of AIDS will become relevant considerations on the subject of the damages that can be recovered.

In addition to the theory of negligent transmission of AIDS, there also are other theories that plaintiffs can assert. These include, at a minimum, battery, fraud, and intentional infliction of emotional distress. The action for battery for sexually transmitted diseases has been allowed under the view that while the plaintiff consents to the sexual touching, the plaintiff does not consent to exposure to an infectious condition. Actions for fraud and intentional infliction of emotional distress have been allowed in cases involving sexually transmitted diseases where the defendant knew of his or her infection and concealed or withheld knowledge about the infection from the plaintiff. *Plaza v. Estate of Wisser*.

The best known case involving the fear of sexual transmission of AIDS is the one brought by Mark Christian against the estate of the late actor Rock

Hudson. Christian sued Hudson's estate on the ground that Hudson knew he had AIDS, concealed his condition from Christian, and continued their sexual relationship. The jury returned a multi-million dollar verdict in favor of Christian despite the fact that there was no evidence that Christian had become infected with HIV.

It should be carefully noted that defendants who can prove that they did not know and had no reason to suspect that they had AIDS will not be held liable when it is later determined that they have passed their HIV infection to others through sexual relations. In *C.A.U. v. R.L.*, for example, the Minnesota Court of Appeals affirmed a trial court's finding that the plaintiff could not recover damages from her former fiance from whom she had contracted AIDS. The court concluded that at the time of the parties' sexual relationship in 1985, the defendant had no reason to suspect that he either had AIDS or was capable of transmitting the virus through sex. Similarly, in *Doe v. Johnson*, basketball star Magic Johnson was sued for sexual transmission of HIV to one of his female sexual partners. The federal trial court held that he had no legal duty to warn his sexual partners where he did not know that he was HIV-infected and where he had merely been promiscuous.

An important practical point about HIV sexual transmission cases concerns the monetary status of the defendant. Ordinarily, defendants will not be in the financial position of a famous actor, such as Rock Hudson, or a star athlete, such as Magic

Johnson. More often, the defendant will have little or no money due to the fact that AIDS regularly bankrupts its victims. Therefore, plaintiffs normally will have to seek out other sources for recovery. One such source may be the proceeds of an apartment dweller's, homeowner's, or automobile owner's insurance policy. If the act of sexual transmission of AIDS occurred in the defendant's residence or car, the defendant's liability policy may cover the injury. To avoid such liability, insurance companies now routinely include in such policies exclusions for sexually transmitted diseases or viral conditions.

Plaintiffs also may attempt to find some other defendant, such as the physician or psychiatrist who cared for the defendant, who knew of the plaintiff's intimate relationship with the defendant and failed to warn the plaintiff of the risk of sexual transmission of AIDS. In a California case, a doctor had failed to disclose the HIV infection of a minor to either the minor or her parents. A few years later the minor began dating and allegedly passed HIV to her boyfriend. The court allowed a cause of action by the boyfriend to proceed against the doctor. *Reisner v. University of California.*

Finally, the right of prisoners to engage in conjugal visits with their families must be considered. In some prisons, inmates are allowed to spend private time alone with their spouses and children. This time often includes an overnight visit in a private separate facility, such as a mobile home or trailer on the prison grounds. Of course, the assumption behind such visits is that they provide prisoners with an opportunity to carry on sexual relationships with their spouses. If prisoners have AIDS, the question arises whether they should be allowed to engage in a conjugal visit with their spouses. The same type of question is present if it is the spouse who is infected. Other questions that may arise include whether a prisoner with AIDS should be allowed to engage in a conjugal visit with a spouse who has AIDS and whether prison officials should be permitted to test prisoners and their spouses for HIV in connection with the administration of conjugal visit programs.

The only reported case in this area is *Doe v. Coughlin*. In that case, the New York State Court of Appeals denied a prisoner with AIDS the right to have a conjugal visit with his wife. After the prisoner had qualified for the family visitation program and had engaged in a private conjugal visit with his wife, he was diagnosed as having AIDS. Although both he and his wife were informed of his AIDS condition, they applied for another conjugal visit. When the prison administration denied their request, they sued to have the decision overturned.

On appeal, the court emphasized that there is no constitutional right to a family visit while in prison and that the only issue is whether there is a rational basis for the prison administration's decision to deny the request. The court found no difficulty in validating the prison's concern that the wife be protected from the possible transmission of HIV. In contrast, the dissenting judges took the view that the protection of a non-prisoner does not serve any proper penological purpose. The dissenters also felt that a wife should be allowed to decide on her own whether to take advantage of a conjugal visit, including what activities to engage in with her husband during the privacy of such a visit. Subsequently, prison administrators announced that they were reversing their policy.

A number of other questions involving conjugal visits and AIDS have yet to be tested in court. If, for example, the spouses promise not to engage in sexual activity or promise to use protective measures such as condoms during sexual intercourse, should conjugal visitation be allowed? Similarly, should conjugal visitation be expanded to allow participation by unmarried heterosexual lovers and by gay and lesbian partners? Finally, can the confidentiality of sensitive information about inmates, their spouses, and AIDS be adequately assured in the prison setting?

C. PARENTING

1. Conception

AIDS has further complicated the already important and difficult decision of whether to have children. The conscious decision of individuals to engage in sexual relations or to utilize artificial insemination or surrogate mothering for the purpose of conceiving a child can result in transmission of HIV if one of the sexual partners, the semen donor, or the surrogate mother is infected.

Medical evidence has established that about 30% of all children born to HIV-infected mothers will contract the virus (although the prophylactic administration of AZT during pregnancy can dramatically reduce the transmission rate). It is not certain whether the transmission occurs during pregnancy or upon birth (prior to the time that the umbilical cord is severed). Furthermore, the mother can pass the virus to a newborn through breast feeding.

The AIDS epidemic has caused particular complications for gay men who wish to father children of their own. Research indicates that there are a large number of gay fathers. Although there has been considerable reluctance on the part of society and the law to approve of gay parenting, many courts had begun to chip away at this view in the years immediately before AIDS. Now, however, there is an aura of doubt about the health and life expectancy of gay men. Many gays are afraid they have HIV or AIDS, while others fear they will seroconvert or become infected. Hence, many gay men are reluctant to donate sperm or engage in sexual intercourse for the purpose of conceiving a child. They fear that if they are infected they may transmit the virus to the mother and the child. They also fear that if they do father a child they may subsequently fall ill and at some point be unable to support and care for the child. Yet another concern is that the children will have to endure the stress and trauma of seeing their parents suffer long, painful deaths.

If an unborn child is at risk of acquiring AIDS because one or both parents have AIDS or are at risk, there will be pressure on the parent or parents to abort the child. In states that have statutes that criminalize the knowing transmission or attempted transmission of HIV, there may be a very real incentive for the parent or parents to seek an abortion to avoid commission of a felony.

2. Adoption

The AIDS epidemic has resulted in substantial complications regarding the adoption of minors. First, the odds are significant that the parent or parents of an HIV-infected child will not wish or will be unable to take and properly care for the child. Many children with HIV or AIDS are abandoned by their parents (or by their mothers in the case of unwed mothers). The mother often is so ill and so racked with emotional and psychological distress due to her own condition and her guilt for bringing a helpless infant into the world to suffer and die from AIDS that she is not in a position to raise the child. Additionally, such mothers often are victims of both poverty and drug addiction.

If the infected infant lives long enough to leave the hospital after birth, it naturally will be quite difficult to find an appropriate placement for such a baby. Few foster care families and even fewer prospective adoptive parents are willing to take in a child where it is known that the child will become progressively debilitated, suffer pain, experience costly medical care needs, and die prematurely in a few months or a few years.

Second, there is the serious problem of the health of the prospective parent or parents of children who might be adopted. An appropriate consideration in the context of any adoption of a minor is the health, both present and long term, of the prospective parent or parents. Assurances are needed that they will be healthy enough to be able to support and care for the child until he or she reaches the age of majority and is self-supporting. On the matter of the appropriateness of a particular adoption decision or placement, the overriding concern of the agencies and the courts is always the best interests of the child. *In re Adoption of Johnson.*

Finally, it should be noted that a number of lawsuits have been filed around the country by adoptive parents against adoption agencies as well as the natural parents of adopted children where there has been concealment of a serious health or emotional problem of the child. Given the critical nature of AIDS, it can be expected that the failure of the natural parents or the adoption agency to disclose that the child is at increased risk for HIV or has HIV infection will result in lawsuits by the adoptive parents. Even this particular area is very complicated, in part because of the medical fact that the HIV antibody status of a newborn actually reflects the antibody status of its mother for a period of between ten and eighteen months after birth. Only after such time is the infant's own immune system sufficiently developed to produce antibody reactions that can be accurately reflected through testing.

3. Children With AIDS

The number of infants and adolescents with AIDS is growing dramatically. Unfortunately, youngsters constitute the largest category of individuals experiencing new infections of HIV.

There is a serious problem in many major metropolitan areas of this country of newborn babies being infected with HIV. The primary route to these newborn children is transmission from an infected mother who acquired AIDS due to intravenous drug use or sexual contact with intravenous drug users. These babies tend to face short, lonely, and painful lives. Many of them are abandoned in the hospitals where they are born. Few ever leave the hospital. Most newborn children do not do well against HIV because their immune systems are not fully developed and because their health is generally unsatisfactory due to a lack of appropriate maternal and prenatal care. Some local hospitals are being overwhelmed by this problem and are running out of bed space for the growing numbers of infants with AIDS.

Adolescents and teenagers also are a group with an increasing AIDS problem. Young people tend to be curious, rambunctious, and daring. They lack the experience and wisdom of older people and may be inclined to experiment with sex and drugs. In an era of AIDS, that can be a deadly combination of factors.

Thus, AIDS education for the purpose of preventing transmission is critical for prospective mothers and children. Education of prospective mothers in hospitals, clinic prenatal care units, schools, and community shelters is essential to curb transmission to newborn children. Young children and adolescents also need information about the risks of AIDS transmission through sexual intercourse and intravenous drug use. Once again, schools and community-based organizations (such as churches, libraries, and park districts) can serve as effective sources of such education.

Parents who transmit AIDS to their newborn children may well be the targets of lawsuits. First, parents may be the subjects of criminal prosecutions under the statutes in many states that criminalize the knowing transmission of HIV. Indeed, knowingly transmitting AIDS to a newborn might even be prosecuted as a criminal offense under general criminal statutes, such as those dealing with attempted murder and reckless conduct. Second, parents may be subject to a lawsuit by the state to terminate their parental rights if they knowingly permit the transmission of AIDS to their children. It would certainly seem that such conduct by a parent would constitute parental neglect and endangerment of the health of their children. State agencies have sought to terminate the parental rights of drug-abusing parents whose newborn children are adversely affected by such drugs. Third, parents who knowingly transmit AIDS to their children may be subject to tort actions filed on behalf of the children. Lawsuits have been sustained on behalf of infants against their mothers for injuries suffered by the children while *in utero* due to the negligence of the mothers.

D. SEPARATION AND DIVORCE

1. Break-Up of Relationships

Although the AIDS epidemic has contributed to couples getting together and staying together, it also has led to the break-up of couples. Even in the best of circumstances personal relationships are difficult to maintain, and the presence of AIDS as well as the fear of AIDS can make matters even more difficult.

If one of the parties to a relationship has AIDS, both parties will encounter concerns about how and when the virus was transmitted. The infected party may experience guilt, depression, anger, and lethargy. The other individual may feel betrayed, uncertain, fearful, and hostile. The party with AIDS has the prospect of needing substantial medical care, of becoming progressively less able to care for himself or herself, and of dying an early and perhaps agonizing death. Even where neither of the parties to a relationship has AIDS, one individual may fear or suspect the other. If one party believes that the other is guilty of infidelity (such as having needle-sharing or sexual relationships outside the marital or cohabitation arrangement), serious obstacles to a harmonious relationship can arise.

Where a marriage is involved, it may be possible to have the marriage annulled or to obtain a divorce. Among the well-established bases for the annulment of a marriage are situations in which a party has been duped into marriage by a fraud involving the essentials of marriage or where a party lacks the physical capacity to consummate the marriage by sexual intercourse and the other party does not know of the incapacity. Although it is clear that individuals do not have a duty to know their AIDS status, once they do learn that they are infected with HIV they have a responsibility to either refrain from risky activity or to inform their sexual partners prior to engaging in sex. Thus, there is a duty to inform a prospective spouse where an individual knows that he or she has AIDS. The failure of one party to advise the other about one's AIDS condition amounts to fraud going to the essentials of marriage, and an individual with AIDS would be unable to consummate the marriage through unprotected sexual relations because of the risk of transmitting an incurable, fatal condition to the other partner (since the other partner would not have been informed of the condition and would not have consented to sexual intercourse with such knowledge).

The fact that a spouse is infected with AIDS may also serve as the basis for the other spouse obtaining a divorce. If a spouse contracts AIDS subsequent to the marriage, either through adultery or through the use of intravenous drugs, the uninfected spouse can seek a divorce. The reason for this is not the AIDS condition itself, but rather the adultery or the use of addictive drugs. The divorce laws ordinarily list adultery and addiction to drugs as bases for divorce. Further, the divorce statutes commonly provide that if one spouse has attempted to take the life of the other or has infected the other with a communicable venereal disease, such circumstances will serve as grounds for a divorce. If a spouse who knows that he or she has AIDS engages in sex or the sharing of intravenous drug needles with the other spouse, there has been an assault of a life-threatening nature upon the other spouse and there may have been infection with a communicable disease that may be regarded as a venereal disease. Many states now have statutes that criminalize the knowing exposure to, or transmission of, AIDS through sexual intercourse and the sharing of intravenous drug needles, and felony prosecutions for attempted murder have been brought in several states resulting from the attempted transmission of AIDS through other activities.

2. Child Custody and Visitation

In divorce cases where minor children are involved, the parents' battle to win custody of or visitation with the children can be quite fierce and can result in severe emotional problems in the children. AIDS impacts on this aspect of the law because the issue of the health of both the children and the parents must be considered. As always, the law takes the position that the best interests of the children should guide decisions relating to custody and visitation.

In the early days of the AIDS epidemic, there was a greater tendency for one parent to panic and to assert or threaten to assert the possible AIDS condition of the other parent. A few judges fell prey to such hysteria and ordered parents, especially gay fathers, to submit to HIV testing as a prerequisite to the awarding of child custody or visitation rights.

There are two leading cases, one on child custody and one on child visitation, that establish that the AIDS condition of a parent cannot serve as the sole basis for terminating or disallowing custody or visitation by that parent. In *Doe v. Roe,* a New York state trial court refused to require a gay father suspected of having AIDS to submit to an HIV test as a precondition to continued custody of his children. The court emphasized the lack of medical evidence that the father would present any health risk to the children, the unreliability of HIV test results in some circumstances, and the severe emotional stress that would be placed upon the father if he were required to be tested and were found to be HIV positive.

In *Stewart v. Stewart,* an Indiana state trial court terminated the visitation rights of a father who had tested positive for HIV. Both the trial judge and the dissenting judge on appeal accepted the view that even if there was only a slight possibility that the child might be exposed to AIDS, the father should be barred from visitation with the infant.

The appellate court majority reversed due to its finding that the medical evidence showed that AIDS is not transmitted through everyday household contacts.

These cases should firmly put to rest the notion that the AIDS status of a parent by itself bars custody or visitation with minor children. Nevertheless, in a case presenting circumstances indicating that the health or well-being of the child would be jeopardized by custody or visitation with an HIV-infected parent, such custody or visitation will be denied or restricted. Thus, for example, it is possible that a parent might, because of AIDS, become physically incapable of properly caring for a child. Similarly, the parent might suffer AIDS-related dementia or emotional distress and be unable to properly care for the child. A parent suffering from AIDS also could become financially unable to have custody of a child. In all of these circumstances, AIDS will likely be relevant to decisions about custody and visitation.

E. ESTATE PLANNING

1. Death and Dying With AIDS

A brief review of some of the medical aspects of AIDS is appropriate in the context of estate planning issues. Although there are a wide variety of individualized conditions encountered by persons living with AIDS, there are a number of common events that occur and affect directly concerns about estate planning. For example, many individuals with AIDS ultimately suffer great physical incapacity, including blindness. These individuals cannot get out and about to do the simplest tasks, such as shopping, cashing a check, visiting a bank, or getting to a health care facility. AIDS is a terribly expensive disease that often bankrupts its victims. As medical science has succeeded in more effectively treating the symptoms of AIDS, it has prolonged the lives of people with AIDS. This has increased the costs associated with the illness. Finally, severe emotional distress and dementia are a fact of life for many people struggling with AIDS. These conditions may render some individuals mentally incapable of making financial and health care decisions. Indeed, there is a great deal of evidence that suggests that suicide is an increasing occurrence among people with AIDS.

Early and thorough estate planning can provide an important means by which to reduce the substantial burden on the family and friends of one who is dying of AIDS. Proper estate planning is also an important emotional tool by which those struggling with AIDS can exert some control over their own lives. AIDS otherwise saps individuals of such control, for it takes away their health, their finances, their relationships with family and friends, and, finally, their lives. A proper estate plan can provide individuals with the opportunity to make important determinations about their finances and about their health and medical care. It also can provide an individual with the power to determine how certain things will happen even after he or she dies (such as the disposition of one's body and property).

Many people with AIDS who have life insurance now have the option to enter into viatical settlements (*i.e.*, to cash-out their policies). This alternative should be considered in connection with financial planning for individuals with AIDS, along with all of the other possible sources of financial support for the costs of medical care, housing, living expenses, and funeral arrangements.

For those people with AIDS who live in non-traditional relationships, a thorough and thoughtful estate plan serves as a means for providing for the members of the non-traditional family. Although the law may not recognize a same-sex marriage, the law will quite readily allow one partner to give a same-sex partner a power of attorney to make medical and financial decisions and will permit the disposition of the property of the deceased to a same-sex partner. Thus, with respect to some of the practical issues relevant to the process of dying and death, particularly disposal of the property of the decedent, there is less of a need to legitimize or formalize the "family" relationship.

Many states now have health care surrogate decisionmaking statutes that permit someone else to make a patient's critical health and medical care decisions (including decisions not to undertake, or to discontinue, extraordinary life support measures) when the patient has become mentally incompetent to do so. These statutes apply only when a patient's condition has become hopeless, such as where the patient is in a terminal condition or in a persistent comatose condition from which there is no prospect of recovery. Moreover, the statutes apply only where the patient has not executed an effective advance medical directive of some kind, such as a living will or durable power of attorney.

These surrogate decisionmaking laws establish a hierarchy of individuals who can make critical medical care decisions on behalf of the patient. The list of surrogates commonly places the patient's spouse or guardian at the top of the list and the patient's close blood or adoptive relatives next in priority. Usually, close friends appear near the end of the list of surrogates. Almost none of the surrogate laws separately include a domestic partner or significant other on their list.

2. Durable Powers of Attorney, Living Wills, and Wills and Trusts

Due in part to developments with regard to the AIDS epidemic, a number of states have adopted special statutory provisions for durable powers of attorney and living wills. These devices are intended to supplement the more traditional estate planning devices of wills and trusts. In these days of advancing medical technology, even people who are not at risk for AIDS should consider completing these documents, especially in light of the recognition accorded to them by the United States Supreme Court in *Cruzan v. Missouri Department of Health.*

A durable power of attorney is a form of agency granted by an individual to someone to act on his or her behalf regarding financial and business dealings. It is intended to last for a period of time and is not affected by the subsequent physical or mental incapacity of the grantor. As suggested earlier, individuals with AIDS may well encounter a time when they cannot engage in the simplest of activities, let alone care for their business and financial matters. It is important to have someone who can undertake such activities and make decisions when the principal is unable to do so.

A living will is a device by which an individual can decide about possible future medical and health care decisions. Importantly, the living will provides a way for individuals to designate in advance whether they wish to be cared for or sustained by extraordinary lifesaving medical efforts. The living will also can provide a means by which to make decisions about who can visit the individual with AIDS and which health professionals will provide care. Although these are the common distinctions between a durable power of attorney and a living will, the law in the particular state in question must be consulted because specific state statutes normally have one or more unique provisions and the characteristics of the two devices may overlap in certain jurisdictions.

Just as traditional estate planning instruments such as wills and trusts can be challenged, so too can there be challenges to durable powers of attorney and living wills. Sometimes the members of the blood family of an individual with AIDS will attempt to attack these instruments if authority has been granted to someone outside the traditional family. Similarly, a member of a non-traditional family might challenge a durable power of attorney, a living will, or a will or trust if some power or property has been given to members of the traditional family.

In the context of AIDS, the two key challenges that can be leveled against these instruments are the incapacity of the individual with AIDS to execute such documents and the undue influence of others in pressuring the individual with AIDS into executing the instruments. The validity of an instrument may be attacked on the basis that the individual who executed it lacked the mental capacity to do so. Because AIDS is an incurable and fatal condition, individuals who live with the illness suffer from a great deal of stress and psychological pressure. Full-scale dementia is a result for some people with AIDS. The question then is either the "contract standard" of whether the individual understood in a reasonable manner the nature and consequences of his or her transactions, or the "testamentary standard" which involves a lower level of capacity, as discussed in *Bober v. Harrison*. The answer to the inquiry will depend upon the facts of a particular case, which often requires the court to recite and consider the circumstances in great detail, as was done in *Estate of Wilford*.

The validity of an instrument also is subject to challenge on the basis that it was the result of undue influence exerted by some other party. In order for the undue influence argument to prevail, it must be established that the person with AIDS was in a position in which he or she was vulnerable to outside pressure and that the other party was in an opportune position to take advantage of the circumstances. An individual with AIDS may well be vulnerable to another's influence. Persons with AIDS may suffer from some degree of diminished capacity (be it physical, emotional, or mental), and as the disease progresses their vulnerability may increase. Furthermore, the people around an individual living with AIDS may well enjoy a special relationship that provides the opportunity to unduly influence or take advantage of the circumstances. Especially in the case of a non-traditional relationship, the partner will occupy such a close position to the individual with AIDS that an appearance of impropriety may readily be created. That is what happened in *In re Thaler*, where the court considered both issues of incapacity and undue influence and upheld the will.

For all of the foregoing reasons, the preparation and execution of instruments such as durable powers of attorney, living wills, and wills and trusts needs to be done with care and caution to assure that they are not subject to challenge on the grounds of incapacity or undue influence. These documents should be prepared as early as possible, at a time when the individual executing them is less likely to be suffering from incapacity and is therefore less likely to be subject to the undue influence of others. The party executing the documents should be queried at each stage to assure counsel and witnesses that the individual has capacity and is not the victim of undue influence. Counsel should also consider videotaping the execution ceremony, so as to have additional proof of capacity.

F. FINAL ARRANGEMENTS

1. Disposition of the Body and Funeral Ceremonies

A surprising number of disputes can arise in connection with the arrangements and conduct of a funeral after the death of someone with AIDS. These problems can include a wide range of matters. What funeral home should be retained to conduct the services? Will the decedent be cremated or buried in the more usual fashion? Who will be allowed to attend the funeral? How will the services be paid for?

Especially where a non-traditional relationship is involved, the funeral may be the time that is ripe for a major confrontation with the blood family. The natural family may wish to exclude the non-traditional partner, or vice versa. The wishes of the decedent may not be honored, especially if they have not been written down or otherwise recorded. Because time is short, there are serious practical difficulties in attempting to resolve a dispute by means of protracted legal proceedings. It therefore is important for the decedent either to have left clear instructions with regard to such matters as the conduct of the funeral or to have made a clear designation regarding who has the authority to make decisions about funeral arrangements. Where funeral arrangements have been made with a particular funeral home and have been pre-paid in whole or in part, there may be some reluctance on the part of both traditional and non-traditional family members to object.

In *Clarke v. Reilly*, the decedent, who had succumbed to complications caused by AIDS, had made it clear to friends and medical staff that he wished to be cremated, to have his ashes placed in a favorite rose coffee pot, and to have the pot given to his long-time male partner. He insisted that he not be buried and that his blood family (from whom he had been estranged for a decade) not be informed of his death. Upon his death, his mother intervened, took control of the body and the funeral arrangements, had the body cremated, and had the ashes buried. When his partner sued, the court ordered the ashes to be exhumed and turned over to the partner in order to carry out the decedent's wishes.

There have been instances where funeral homes have refused to perform services for people with AIDS. Such refusals undoubtedly stem from unwarranted fear of transmission of AIDS or from a concern that other customers will be disinclined to use the services of a funeral home that caters to people with AIDS. Some legal proceedings have been instituted against funeral homes that have refused to provide services for persons who have died of AIDS, but this does not seem to be much of a recurring problem, especially in more recent times as information about AIDS has become more widely disseminated.

2. Death Certificates and Obituaries

Because there has been so much hysteria and unwarranted discrimination associated with persons with AIDS, even the preparation of death certificates and obituaries has been cause for concern for both the surviving family and friends of the decedent. If the death certificate or obituary identifies the cause of death as complications from AIDS, family and friends of the decedent may well suffer from their association with the decedent. Other people may assume that the family and friends have AIDS or are at increased risk for AIDS.

As a result, there has been great variation in the preparation of death certificates and obituaries. Since people do not die of AIDS itself, but rather from one of the opportunistic diseases that can more freely invade the body of a person whose immune system is depressed, both death certificates and obituaries can readily be written without any direct reference to AIDS. While some death certificates and obituaries refer very directly to AIDS, others make no such references and report the cause of death as pneumonia, cancer, or some other general cause. Again, it is probably the case that if the individual with AIDS prepares her or his obituary for later use, there will be reluctance on the part of family or friends to amend its contents.

CHAPTER IV

INSURANCE LAW

A. INTRODUCTION

The AIDS epidemic appeared at a time when the system of financing health care in the United States was in considerable flux. Unlike most industrialized Western countries, the United States does not have a national health insurance system. Instead, there are a variety of public programs dealing with particular defined population groups (such as the poor, the elderly, and the disabled). Those who do not qualify for such programs are left to secure their own financing for health care, which is accomplished through the purchase of insurance, as a benefit of employment, or by direct cash payment as the need arises. AIDS has generated a multitude of issues within the health finance system. Some issues cut across the different financing mechanisms, while others are peculiar to the particular mechanism under discussion.

This chapter will not consider issues raised by life insurance or other insurance programs that do not relate directly to payment for health care. As to life insurance, in particular, there is general agreement among the states that life insurers may impose HIV testing requirements and disqualify infected persons from purchasing life insurance, provided they comply with any applicable state laws requiring informed consent and other procedural safeguards (including confidentiality of test results).

B. HISTORICAL BACKGROUND

Prior to the 20th century, individuals financed their own health care through personal arrangements with doctors and hospitals. Those too poor to pay for their own care fell back on charity hospitals (which were frequently connected to religious organizations) or the kindness of individual doctors who provided a certain amount of free care as a professional moral obligation. In an age without miracle drugs or cures for most infectious diseases, health care was cheap but also relatively ineffective. Those whose medical difficulties could be shown to be caused by the intentional or negligent conduct of others might recover the costs of treatment through the torts system, although late 19th century tort law developed various doctrines that shielded employers—the most likely sources of financing—from having to pay the medical expenses for most of the work-related injuries of their employees.

The development of modern medicine has changed all this. Besides making health care quite expensive but also considerably more effective, the issue of financing care is now a major preoccupation of society. The health insurance industry we know today is largely a 20th century invention, following on legislative reform of tort law that established a social insurance system (called workers' compensation) to deal with some of the costs of work-related injuries. Employment-related health insurance largely grew out of collective bargaining during World War II, when government-imposed wage controls precluded unions from demanding direct wage increases. The rapid adoption of health insurance as a standard fringe benefit in unionized companies prodded many non-union companies to offer insurance in order to be competitive in the skilled labor market. Simultaneously, the Blue Cross movement of non-profit health insurance, organized by the medical profession itself, arose with the goal of providing affordable health insurance for individuals and groups. The private, for-profit insurance industry also began to develop health insurance policies for sale to employers, membership associations (such as associations of self-employed professionals like lawyers and doctors), unions, and individuals.

At the same time, beginning in the 1930s, the federal government began to become actively involved in financing the health care of particular population groups. Some of the most important government programs include Medicare, which provides insurance coverage for the elderly and the permanently disabled, and Medicaid, which provides coverage for the poor. In addition, the federal government and many states have established programs to held fund care for particular diseases.

Federal legislation enacted during the early 1970s, known as the Employee Retirement Income Security Act (ERISA), 29 U.S.C.A. §§ 1001 *et seq.*, had a major impact on the structure of the health insurance industry. ERISA created a federal scheme for regulating employee benefit plans and largely preempted the states and localities from regulating such plans. However, ERISA did not itself impose many substantive requirements on health insurance plans, being primarily concerned with the details of pension regulation. At the same time, ERISA largely left in place the traditional role of the states as the primary regulators of the health insurance industry (despite the emergence of large national health insurance companies that had come to dominate the industry by that time). ERISA's preemption of state and local regulation was thus incomplete, because ERISA expressly preserved the states' ability to regulate insurance companies.

The net result of this enactment, as it worked out over the next two decades, was to give larger employers a strong incentive to terminate their arrangements with insurance companies and instead directly fund the health care benefits of their employees. Early court decisions determined that such "self-insurance" schemes were sheltered from state and local regulation by ERISA; by contrast, when an employer provided health benefits to employees by purchasing a group health insurance policy from an insurance company, the state could regulate the transaction through its direct regulation of the insurance companies. By establishing self-insured plans, many large employers preserved their flexibility to design and administer benefits without the interference of state regulators. Because neither Congress nor federal administrators made any effort to impose substantive rules on self-insured employers, their health benefit plans were essentially unregulated as to coverage and scope, apart from an ERISA provision ostensibly forbidding any discrimination by employers that would prevent employees from receiving benefits to which they were entitled under the plans. By the mid–1980s, most large employers were "self-insured" and the trend was toward self-insurance for moderate-sized employers as well.

At the same time, rising insurance company premiums led many small employers to abandon health benefit programs entirely. By the beginning of the 1990s, it was estimated that more than one-third of the workforce had no health insurance coverage, and the press was full of stories about uninsured families who had to spend down to poverty levels in order to qualify for Medicaid to finance ongoing treatment of chronic illnesses. In the 1992 national elections, health care financing was a major issue in the presidential race and many congressional races. However, the complicated health care reform plan subsequently proposed by the Clinton Administration drew immediate opposition from the private insurance industry as well as many members of Congress. As a result, attempts to radically change the system stalled.

The election of Republican majorities in both the House and Senate in 1994 appears to have doomed systemic health care reform for the immediate future. On the other hand, in 1995 Congressional Republicans proposed significant changes in the funding mechanisms for federal-sponsored insurance systems that would, for the first time, abandon the concept of federal entitlements and delegate to the states a significant share of the responsibility for allocating limited funds for health care.

C. BASIC PRINCIPLES OF INSURANCE FUNDING

Health insurance is structured according to principles of actuarial science, which is the science of calculating and funding risks. The insurance system is supposed to make health care affordable for individuals by spreading the risk over such large population groups that the cost to individual participants is manageable. By studying the actual experience of a given population, an actuary can calculate the likelihood of particular events occurring in that population in the future and the level of funding that will be necessary to cover the resulting medical costs. In the for-profit sector, insurers establish payment requirements (called "premiums") that will fund a pool of money sufficient to cover claims by the insurance policy purchasers while returning a profit to the company through earnings made by investing the funds.

Thus, to take a crude example, if the likelihood of a heart attack occurring in a particular population group is one a year for one hundred people, and an insurance policy was intended to just cover heart attacks, an insurer could set individual premiums such that they would generate a fund large enough to cover the costs attributable to one heart attack per year, while leaving enough additional money invested to cover the insurance company's administrative expenses and generate a profit for its shareholders after paying corporate taxes to the government.

In the not-for-profit sector, meaning, primarily, Blue Cross and Blue Shield, premiums can theoretically be set lower because there is no need to generate a profit for shareholders of the company, and because, as a not-for-profit enterprise, the provider may benefit from preferential tax treatment for its income. Government health insurance plans are also funded according to actuarial principles, although the funding sources are different from the private sector (but not entirely, as elderly Medicare participants are required to pay premiums for coverage).

In order to implement the findings of the actuaries, insurance companies have traditionally devised methods to ensure that the actual benefit claims they receive are consistent with actuarial calculations based on past claims. These methods focus both on preventing the purchase of insurance by persons who would predictably increase the risk of claims in the insured population, and on avoiding liability for claims by insured individuals either through strict interpretations of restrictive coverage terms in insurance contracts, by cancellation of policies, or by inclusion of provisions that deny coverage for medical conditions that existed before the insured purchased the policy.

The AIDS epidemic, as a new phenomenon of the early 1980s, was not anticipated by the insurance industry and not factored into the actuarial calculations the industry used to set premiums. As a result, the first impulse of many insurers was to attempt to avoid paying claims for HIV-related treatment or to treat HIV-infection that may have predated purchase of the policy as a "pre-existing condition" excluded from coverage under the policy's terms. Most of the legal developments concerning financing of AIDS care involve efforts by insurers to limit or escape liability or efforts by persons with AIDS to obtain coverage to which they feel entitled under insurance plans. The balance of this chapter will examine the legal issues brought to light by this litigation.

D. ACCESS TO INSURANCE

At the beginning of the AIDS epidemic, most insurance companies did not conduct an individual evaluation of the potential risk of insuring individuals under group policies unless the group was very small. For small groups and individual policy applicants, the companies undertook a process called "underwriting," by which the insurer sought to determine whether the applicant would present an "unacceptable" risk. Underwriting was concerned with identifying "risk factors" associated with the likelihood of future claims, such as current health status, family medical history, smoking habits, and similar concerns. Government health plans and most not-for-profit plans did not require individual underwriting.

In the context of AIDS, as soon as it became clear to insurance companies that unanticipated claims for very expensive hospitalizations were being presented from an identifiable group of insureds (primarily gay white men), insurance companies began to undertake efforts to use the underwriting process to avoid adding such individuals to their insured populations. The most straightforward method was to add a question to the standard application form, asking if the applicant had experienced any AIDS symptoms or been diagnosed with AIDS. Since health insurance application forms typically contain such questions with respect to a wide variety of medical conditions, the addition of AIDS to the list seemed appropriate in the context of standard underwriting. In cases such as *Sapp v. Paul Revere Life Ins. Co.* and *Espinosa v. Guardian Life Ins.*, the courts have held that insurance applicants who conceal knowledge about their AIDS status can later be denied benefits for HIV-related claims.

Some companies, realizing from epidemiological data that particular population groups appeared more likely to develop AIDS, have undertaken less straightforward methods of eliminating AIDS risk, such as by adopting informal standards that would exclude suspected members of AIDS "risk groups" on the basis of stereotypical demographic factors. For example, in one case an insurance company, citing "blood irregularities" in a test performed prior to the availability of screening tests for HIV, turned down an application for health insurance from an unmarried male law student living in New York City with another unmarried man. The applicant sued, claiming an unfair insurance practice under state law. Faced with bad publicity, the insurance company settled the case. Clearly, the attempt was being made to avoid adding a gay man to the insurance pool. Ironically, the student was not gay.

In other instances, documented on the West Coast by National Gay Rights Advocates, a now defunct public interest law firm, insurance companies tried to avoid selling group policies to employers in industries believed to have a heavy representation of gay male employees. Such "redlining" violated California insurance laws, and several companies settled discrimination claims by promising to refrain from such underwriting practices.

The effort to escape AIDS liability through underwriting advanced to a more sophisticated stage when the FDA licensed the ELISA screening test for HIV antibodies in 1985. Soon health insurance companies began to require HIV testing of applicants. Those advocating against the exclusion of people at risk for AIDS from the general insured population had two potential courses of action: seek a ban on HIV testing by insurers or argue more broadly against the practice of individual underwriting.

While these advocates were successful in persuading some regulators that banning HIV testing for health insurance underwriting was a good public policy decision, they were less successful with legislators. The advocates argued that allowing the private health insurance industry to test for HIV would, in effect, provide a significant public subsidy to the insurance industry, because uninsurable individuals would eventually present themselves for treatment at public hospitals and seek funding under Medicaid after they had impoverished themselves with medical expenses. In addition, advocates argued that those with private insurance tended to qualify for and receive better treatment, thus preserving their health (and their productive contribution as workers and taxpayers) longer and justifying, as a matter of economics, government efforts to protect their insurability in the private sector.

When regulators in Massachusetts and New York attempted to ban HIV-testing administratively, the insurance industry sued and obtained decisions from the highest courts in both states that such a fundamental change to the underwriting process could not be taken administratively, but instead required actual legislation. In *Life Ins. Ass'n v. Commissioner of Insurance* and *Health Ins. Ass'n of America v. Corcoran*, the courts noted that their state legislatures had authorized insurance companies to engage in individual underwriting practices so long as they did not discriminate by treating people who presented the same risks differently. The courts went on to decide that people with HIV-infection present a significantly different claims risk than people without such infection; consequently, the insurance companies were justified in attempting to identify such individuals and subjecting them to different treatment. As a practical matter, insurance companies were treating HIV-infected people as uninsurable because, especially early in the epidemic, there were no well-established cost figures for treatment from which an appropriate premium could be calculated. If the figures generated by the first few thousand cases were used, the premiums would be so high as to render insurance unaffordable.

It must be remembered that private insurance companies are not organized as charitable institutions; they are businesses that must generate profits for their shareholders if they want to remain in operation. The key policy question before the courts in these cases was whether the legislatively-created principles governing the business of insurance could credibly be interpreted by regulators to require insurers to shoulder the burden of funding AIDS treatment at the same rates they were charging to cover other, actuarially-anticipated, risks. The courts' answer was no.

In other states, legislators were persuaded by the arguments of advocates for people with AIDS to outlaw the use of the HIV test for health insurance underwriting. California, Rhode Island, and Wisconsin were among the first states to do so, although critics contended that the laws in Rhode Island and Wisconsin were ineffective due to loopholes that allowed testing once the HIV test had been demonstrated to be actuarially reliable. The District of Columbia Council also passed a ban on HIV testing by insurers. Although the industry went to court, arguing that requiring it to incur the risks of AIDS treatment without allowing HIV testing was an unconstitutional taking of property, the ban was upheld as a regulatory measure within the authority of the Council. *American Council of Life Insurance v. District of Columbia*. However, the industry's lobbyists then went to work on Congress, which subsequently pressured the Council to rescind its ban.

After the industry won its litigation in New York, the state legislature became more receptive to arguments that allowing individual underwriting was contributing substantially to the rising costs of state and local government-funded health care in the state. It therefore adopted a new law banning individual underwriting for health insurance. As predicted by industry lobbyists, some companies withdrew from the individual health insurance market (as they had in the District of Columbia until Congress forced the city to rescind its HIV testing ban), while others substantially raised their rates in anticipation of a jump in benefits claims as previously uninsurable people purchased policies.

In some states that still allow individual underwriting and the use of HIV tests, those found "uninsurable" are sometimes able to obtain insurance coverage under an assigned-risk program in which insurance companies have agreed to take a certain number of insureds through a state program at inflated premium rates. In other states, they may be able to purchase coverage through a state-operated insurance fund.

Most insurance contracts include a provision, called an incontestability clause, that provides that after a specified period of time has passed—normally two years—the insurance company may not "contest" the validity of the application or seek to cancel or revoke the insurance contract based on faults with the application. In the context of AIDS, the issue has been whether an insurer can defeat a claim for AIDS-related benefits on the basis that the applicant concealed his or her HIV status at the time of the application, knowing or having reason to know that he or she was HIV-positive at the time.

In *Fioretti v. Massachusetts General Life Ins. Co.*, the Eleventh Circuit held that a life insurance policy applicant's deliberate attempts to defeat the insurer's underwriting process by concealing his HIV status and submitting a friend's blood sample to avoid detection provided a valid basis for allowing the insurer to rescind the policy after the insured had died from AIDS and his beneficiary had filed a claim. Although the policy did contain an incontestability clause whose time limit had run out before the claim was filed, the court decided that there was an exception to the normal incontestability rules where it could be shown that the applicant had committed an active fraud against the insurance company. However, in *Amex Life Assurance Co. v. Superior Court,* a California state appellate court enforced an incontestability clause even though the applicant had sent an imposter to take his blood test.

E.   COVERAGE ISSUES

Another mechanism used by the insurance industry to attempt to preserve the risk level in its insured populations is to write exclusionary language into insurance policies. Most often, this language seeks to limit the insurer's liability to medical conditions that occur after the insurance coverage goes into effect (excluding coverage for "pre-existing" conditions), and then only for standardized, well-recognized treatments, and not for treatments deemed "experimental" because they are too new to have an established track record for effectiveness. Since many newer procedures and drugs are very expensive, such an exclusion can be a big money-saver for insurers. However, because AIDS is a new epidemic for which traditional, established treatments are unavailable or ineffective, exclusionary provisions tend to disqualify many treatment regimens from coverage.

The insurance industry is not the only actor in this drama that is attempting to use exclusionary coverage language as a risk avoidance measure. The Medicare and Medicaid programs also eschew coverage for "experimental" treatment. One rationale for such exclusions is that insurance programs, whether in the public or private sector, are established on the basis of actuarial principles designed to spread known risks among the insured populations, and the expense of experimental treatments logically falls outside the sphere of "known risks." Another rationale is that insurers, whether private or public, should not spend the pooled resources of the insured group (or taxpayers' money) on untried treatments that might turn out to be totally ineffective.

The expense of developing new treatments in a capitalist system of private enterprise are theoretically to be borne by those who stand to profit from them—in the case of AIDS, research laboratories and drug companies that stand to profit if they can establish that their products are safe and effective in treating AIDS-related immune deficiency or opportunistic infections. Part of the costs of drug development are clinical trials in which experimental drugs are administered and their safety and effectiveness monitored by researchers. Participants in the trials normally receive the drug for free, so insurance companies are not presented with claims for such experimental treatments. Prior to the advent of AIDS, most experimental treatment claims issues dealt with new surgical procedures, such as organ transplants, and major research hospitals frequently found themselves absorbing the extremely high costs for such procedures until they became routinized enough to satisfy insurers that they were no longer experimental.

AIDS presented new issues, primarily due to the impact on the traditional, slow drug development process of a disease that affected a largely upper-middle class, articulate subpopulation that was able to mobilize political force to upset the traditional system. AIDS activists, through demonstrations, lobbying, and political organizing, were able to secure early approval of some experimental drugs—most notably AZT—for limited specified use. When patients sought to use the drugs in situations not specified in the FDA's official "label" for the drug, insurers tried to refuse payment.

In *Weaver v. Reagen*, the court dealt with such a dispute when the Missouri Medicaid program refused to reimburse patients for AZT used outside the scope of the FDA's original authorization. The Missouri regulations, in line with the FDA label, specified that Medicaid would pay for AZT for persons who met the CDC's definition of full-blown AIDS. Many doctors in Missouri and elsewhere were administering AZT to patients who did not meet the CDC definition, which was widely acknowledged to have lagged behind newer knowledge about the progression of HIV infection. Some studies had shown that people who took AZT at an earlier stage of infection might prolong their period of good health before developing AIDS. But Medicaid refused to pay for the drug, which was much too expensive for most individuals.

The court found that Missouri's refusal to pay for AZT outside the FDA's labelled use violated basic principles of the federal Medicaid program. While the public officials claimed that they had reasonably exercised their discretion to prevent spending public funds on "unapproved" treatments, the court found that determining whether the treatment was covered required looking at the actual practices of doctors who were treating the condition. By the time of the litigation, AZT treatment for HIV-infected people who did not yet meet the CDC's AIDS definition was rapidly becoming "standard" treatment. The court also noted that FDA labelling was never interpreted to impose a limitation on how doctors determined what to prescribe as treatment; as such, it could not be used as the standard to determine whether a treatment was experimental or standard.

To illustrate the point, the court noted that it had previously held, in *Pinneke v. Preisser*, that the Iowa Medicaid program could not refuse to provide coverage for sex reassignment surgery as a treatment for transsexualism, since such surgery had become accepted among physicians as an appropriate treatment, albeit exotic and rare. If Medicaid was required to pay for the occasional sex-change operation, it could not very well refuse to reimburse AIDS patients for AZT treatment.

A more traditional forum for litigating about coverage exclusions, as noted above, focuses on surgical procedures. In the case of AIDS, there was a time in the late 1980s when some doctors were experimenting with bone marrow transplants as a possible means of stimulating the immune system to increase production of the T-cells destroyed by HIV.

Bone marrow transplants had begun to approach the level of widely-accepted treatment in some other illnesses. One of the greatest difficulties, however, was that transplants pose a high risk of rejection of the transplanted tissue by the immune system of the host's body. AIDS researchers hoped to avoid this problem by finding donors who presented very close matches to the genetic composition of the host.

Thomas J. Bradley, a public school teacher in New York with AIDS, had a twin brother who was willing to donate bone marrow. After genetic testing determined that they were identical twins, and that Bradley's health was otherwise good enough to justify risking the operation, they applied for advance approval from Empire Blue Cross and Blue Shield, the provider of group health insurance to the school district in which Bradley was employed. Empire determined that the procedure in the context of AIDS was experimental and thus excluded under the insurance contract. Bradley immediately sought judicial interpretation of the insurance policy.

At trial, the insurance company took the position that a surgical procedure is experimental in the context of a particular disease until controlled studies had shown it to be safe and effective. Bradley introduced an expert who testified about the relatively long history of using the transplant procedure, which had become accepted by the medical community for use with various kinds of illnesses that resembled AIDS in one way or another. The court found that the procedure had become well-enough established to avoid the exclusionary language in the insurance contract, even though the hospital where the procedure was to be performed routinely required patients to sign a "clinical investigation consent form" normally used for experimental procedures. *Bradley v. Empire Blue Cross and Blue Shield.*

Unfortunately, by the time the court granted its preliminary injunction requiring the insurer to pay for the operation, Bradley had developed a new opportunistic infection requiring treatment that disqualified him for the procedure. He subsequently died from AIDS, but the published decision in his case stands ready as a precedent for future litigation over new AIDS-related uses of surgical procedures previously developed in the context of other diseases.

In addition to exclusions of specific treatments, some insurance companies may try to exclude all coverage for HIV-related claims, or declare HIV-infected persons totally uninsurable. The lack of significant litigation about this may indicate that few, if any, insurance companies have pursued this route, probably because state insurance regulators would be likely to challenge such exclusions under fair trade practice laws. In *Anderson v. Gus Mayer Boston Store of Delaware,* a federal district court in Texas found that an employer violated the ADA by purchasing group coverage from an insurer that totally disqualified HIV-infected employees.

On the other hand, some lawsuits have arisen when insurance companies have asserted that AIDS-related claims are barred because the insured was already HIV-infected when the policy was purchased, invoking a "pre-existing condition" clause in the insurance contract. Resolution of such lawsuits will turn on whether a person with HIV infection who has not developed symptoms indicative of CDC-defined AIDS can be said to have a pre-existing condition. Most insurance contracts define a pre-existing condition as a condition known to the applicant for which a reasonable person would have sought medical treatment. Here things may get tricky, since the "state of the art" with HIV infection is to take drugs intended to retard the reproduction of HIV in the bloodstream and as prophylaxis against the possibility of various opportunistic infections; there is considerable division among physicians and people with AIDS, however, about when such a drug regimen should be instituted. Some reasonable people might begin some form of treatment immediately upon learning of their HIV-positive status, while others may believe that treatment should be delayed until a depressed T-cell count triggers more immediate concerns of developing active illness. The issue has yet to be resolved in the courts, although there are precedents from other diseases holding that mere infection without more should not be considered a pre-existing condition. In any event, pre-existing condition clauses normally bar payment for treatment for a specified waiting period, not for the entire duration of the contract, and some states have begun to reform insurance practices by banning such provisions. Proposals to regulate pre-existing condition exclusions were introduced in Congress in 1995.

F. SELF–INSURED EMPLOYERS

As noted above, the combination of federal pre-emption of state laws regulating employee benefit plans and the lack of substantive health plan regulations under ERISA has given employers a strong incentive to fund their health insurance benefits directly rather than purchasing insurance policies (which remain subject to state regulation). Some self-insured employers have sought to take advantage of the lack of direct regulation by placing low life-time caps on HIV-related benefit claims, or by entirely excluding such claims from coverage under their plans. Such exclusions may arise under different scenarios. An employer who is not self-insured may, after learning that employees have submitted claims for HIV-related treatment, convert its health plan to self-insurance and impose a cap or exclusion. Alternatively, an employer who is already self-insured may adopt such a cap or exclusion, either in anticipation of possible HIV-related claims or after such claims have been made on the plan.

Prior to the passage of the ADA, lawyers representing people with AIDS whose employers had imposed caps or exclusions in self-insured plans attempted to gain relief for their clients through federal lawsuits under § 1140 of ERISA, the provision that forbids employers from discriminating against employees for the purpose of depriving them of benefits to which they are entitled. These suits were uniformly unsuccessful.

In the leading case, *McGann v. H & H Music Co.*, the Fifth Circuit ruled that ERISA places no limitation on the flexibility of self-insured employers to adjust their benefit plans, so long as any provisions the employers adopted were uniformly applied to all participants in the plan. John McGann, an H & H Music employee, filed claims for HIV-related treatment at a time when his employer provided health benefits by purchasing a group insurance policy from an insurance company. The insurance policy placed a lifetime cap of $1 million for all claims per employee. Subsequently, the employer switched to self-insurance, preserving the $1 million lifetime cap in general but providing a $5,000 lifetime cap for AIDS-related claims. McGann quickly exhausted this benefit and was denied further reimbursement.

McGann's theory was that by adopting the $5,000 cap after McGann had begun receiving benefits, the employer had discriminated against him for the purpose of depriving him of benefits to which he was entitled. The court disagreed with McGann's theory on two grounds. First, because the cap applied to all employees, and not just McGann, it was not discriminatory. Second, because neither the prior insurance plan nor ERISA imposed any "vesting" requirements for benefits, H & H Music was free to change its benefit plan in response to economic conditions. The court also took note of H & H Music's argument that if it had not taken the steps it did to convert to self-insurance and cap certain kinds of claims, the result might have been complete termination of the benefit. The Eleventh Circuit reached a similar conclusion in *Owens v. Storehouse, Inc.*

With the passage of the ADA, employees with AIDS had a new theory. The employment title of ADA specifically bans discrimination on the basis of disability in the terms and conditions of employment. The EEOC's regulations implementing the discrimination ban construe "terms and conditions of employment" to include "fringe benefits available by virtue of employment, whether or not administered by the [employer.]" However, § 501(c) of the statute, dealing with the impact of the ADA on insurance plans, includes ambiguous language that might be construed as preserving the status quo with respect to health insurance plans. This subsection provides that the ADA should not be construed to "prohibit or restrict" insurers or health maintenance organizations (HMOs) from "underwriting risks, classifying risks, or administering such risks that are based on or not inconsistent with State law" or to "prohibit or restrict" employers or other organizations covered by the ADA from "observing or administering the terms of a bona fide benefit plan that are based on underwriting risks, classifying risks, or administering such risks that are based on or not inconsistent with State law." The subsection also provides that the ADA should not be construed to "prohibit or restrict" employers or other organizations covered by the ADA from "establishing, sponsoring, observing or administering the terms of a bona fide benefit plan that is not subject to State laws that regulate insurance," and concludes that the subsection "shall not be used as a subterfuge to evade the purposes" of the non-discrimination provisions.

On its face, this language suggests that insurance companies and HMOs can continue to engage in underwriting or risk classification in the plans they sell and administer without regard to the impact that the ADA has on employers, and that employers can set up health plans that comply with state laws or that are unregulated by state laws. The language does not affirmatively state that such plans are free of the nondiscrimination requirements of the ADA, and specifically states that the subsection can not be used as a subterfuge for discrimination.

The EEOC took several years after the passage of the ADA to issue its specific interpretation of this language in the context of AIDS caps and exclusions. Finally, it issued a policy statement in 1993 that concluded that caps and exclusions for particular diseases were discriminatory under the ADA, and simultaneously filed suit against some employee benefit plans and employers who were maintaining such caps and exclusions. The issue is in litigation in several district courts, although many of the cases were settled by employers agreeing to remove caps or exclusions and reimburse employees (or their estates) for AIDS-related medical expenses that occurred under the discriminatory policies.

In one of the first decisions to address the principle at issue, the Fourth Circuit ruled that a self-insured employer could not deny coverage to an employee's spouse for expensive chemotherapy by changing the terms of the insurance plan after the insured commenced treatment. *Wheeler v. Dynamic Engineering, Inc.*

G. MAINTAINING COVERAGE

A significant portion of the population obtains health insurance coverage as a benefit of employment. As noted in Chapter 2, if an employee becomes too ill to continue working, an employer may terminate the employment relationship without violating federal, state, or local laws against disability discrimination; only persons with disabilities who are able to perform essential job functions can expect to keep their jobs. While some employers early in the epidemic were willing to keep people with AIDS on their active employee rosters past the time when they could make a productive contribution, in order to preserve their continuing health insurance coverage, other employees were not so lucky. Loss of health insurance coverage was one of the most tragic side-effects of loss of employment, since discharged employees faced significant waiting periods before they could become eligible for Medicaid or permanent disability benefits. Even if a discharged employee could obtain private health insurance (unlikely if underwriting was permitted, since the discharged employee had CDC-defined AIDS), the pre-existing conditions clause would bar payments for AIDS treatment for some substantial period.

Congress addressed these issues by amending ERISA to add provisions creating eligibility for continued participation in employment group health insurance coverage by terminated employees and their dependents. While the former employee participants could be required to bear the costs of premiums to cover their insurance, this overcame the problem of uninsurability faced by discharged employees with AIDS.

H. AIDS AND HEALTH CARE REFORM PROPOSALS

Various proposals that would significantly change the way in which health care is financed in the United States raise significant AIDS policy issues. Reform proposals that emphasize managed care and the use of HMOs to provide coverage for currently uninsured persons might affect the ability of people with AIDS to select and build continuing relationships with appropriate health care providers, unless the reform plans preserve the concept of freedom of choice that prevails under more traditional health insurance programs. Because it has been shown that a patient's chances of receiving effective care are directly tied to his or her physician's knowledge about HIV and AIDS, this is a very important consideration. Moreover, managed care and HMOs are unlikely to provide expansive coverage for new or experimental treatments.

Proposals such as the ones debated in Congress in 1995 to eliminate the traditional Medicaid entitlement system and replace it with block grants to states might lead to rationing of care that would severely affect persons in end-stage AIDS. This possibility is suggested by the rationing system established in the state of Oregon, under which the legislature appropriates a specific level of funding on an annual basis, and medical expenses are covered according to a schedule that ranks treatments in terms of a cost-benefit analysis. Incurable conditions in their final stages are assigned a low priority claim on the finite amount of funds appropriated. Were Congress to abandon the entitlement concept, under which all individuals who meet specified criteria are entitled to the full benefit of Medicaid coverage, in favor of allowing states to decide how to spend their block grants, it would be up to the states to ration the funds they receive.

Those interested in AIDS law will have to pay close attention to health care financing developments to understand how changes in the system may affect the ability of people with AIDS to receive and pay for continuing medical care.

CHAPTER V

CRIMINAL LAW

A. INTRODUCTION

Most health care professionals and public health authorities believe that education and counseling are the best means available to stem transmission of HIV. Evidence suggests that educational programs can be effective in changing the conduct of certain populations at high risk of HIV infection (although there appears to be a decline in the effectiveness of such educational campaigns over time). There is, however, concern that certain individuals, knowing that they are HIV infected, may disregard the risk they pose to others. More disturbingly, certain individuals may deliberately engage in conduct that threatens others with HIV infection. When individuals endanger the health of others by their deliberate or reckless behavior, it has been urged that criminal prosecution should be initiated. And indeed, numerous individuals have been prosecuted and convicted for exposing others to HIV, or, on rare occasions, for actually transmitting HIV to others.

In the context of the AIDS epidemic, there are two kinds of criminal statutes under which HIV-infected persons have been prosecuted for exposing others to HIV or transmitting HIV to others. One type of statute is within the general or traditional criminal law, such as those provisions defining the offenses of attempted murder, battery, and reckless conduct. Such crimes were defined long before AIDS was discovered, and prosecution and conviction require application of old legal doctrines to the more recent circumstances of the danger of transmission of AIDS. The other type of statute is HIV-specific criminal legislation, which was drafted in many states once it became known that AIDS is a transmissible disease.

B. PURPOSES OF CRIMINAL LAW

The purposes underlying the criminal law are realized in appropriate rules and penalties directed at stemming HIV transmission. Those persons who deliberately or recklessly engage in conduct likely to transmit HIV deserve to be punished. In 1988, the *Report of The Presidential Commission on the Human Immunodeficiency Virus Epidemic* stated: "Just as other individuals in society are held responsible for their actions outside the criminal law's established parameters of acceptable behavior, HIV-infected individuals who knowingly conduct themselves in ways that pose a significant risk of transmission to others must be held accountable for their actions." Moreover, there are social reasons to prevent conduct likely to spread HIV. It is thought that criminally prosecuting those who knowingly engage in conduct that risks the spread of HIV will educate the public about conduct likely to spread HIV while at the same time reinforcing social norms against behavior likely to result in HIV transmission.

Serious objections have been raised to the use of the criminal law for prosecution of conduct likely to transmit HIV. Some of these objections can be met easily. Others, however, are compelling and necessitate continued monitoring of both legislative bodies and prosecutorial authorities to prevent violations of civil rights and avoid inappropriate prosecutions.

It may be argued that statutes aimed at controlling behavior intended or likely to spread HIV during sexual activity involve an intrusion into legally protected privacy rights. Courts, however, have refused to recognize the privacy rights of sexual partners as constituting a barrier to criminal convictions arising out of sexual conduct, even in marriage. *State v. Bateman*. Courts in civil cases have held that a constitutional claim of privacy does not preclude an unmarried individual from suing a sexual partner in tort for the sexual transmission of herpes. *Kathleen K. v. Robert B.* The privacy interests of an individual intentionally or knowingly engaging in conduct likely to transmit HIV are similarly outweighed by the social interests in preventing the spread of HIV infection.

It can be argued that criminal laws seeking to prohibit sexual activities between consenting adults do not provide an effective deterrent. The example is cited of the ineffectiveness of sodomy statutes in deterring the behavior they proscribe. There is, however, a difference between a sodomy statute that forbids all sexual activity between partners and an HIV-specific statute, which is directed only to certain behaviors and recognizes a defense based on consent. Such statutes have been enacted in many states.

Some commentators take the view that criminal laws are not effective in deterring HIV-transmitting behavior because such behavior is emotionally charged and irrational. Studies of other forms of sexual behavior, such as incest, however, suggest that statutory schemes that are effectively used to detect, convict, and punish specified sexual behavior can be efficacious.

Because behavior such as unsafe sexual practices and unsafe use of intravenous needles will involve consensual voluntary acts by both parties, an argument can be made that there will be no complaint to legal authorities until there is an indication of HIV infection, which may occur well after the proscribed behavior. Problems of proof resulting from the difference in time between forbidden behavior and awareness of injury may reduce the likelihood of detection and conviction and limit the deterrent effect of any criminal statute. However, it is possible to draft statutory provisions that focus on behavior likely to transmit HIV rather than requiring proof of actual infection. In fact, this is exactly how states have written their HIV-specific criminal laws.

It may be argued that it is unrealistic and inequitable to use the criminal law to discourage behavior related to HIV infection. It has been suggested that it is tantamount to asking individuals to behave at the highest stages of moral development, and it may be unrealistic to expect vulnerable groups, such as drug users or prostitutes, to do so. But if the need to protect others from possible infection might otherwise lead to use of the police power through the public health authority to quarantine or isolate infected individuals, the onus of personal responsibility placed on individuals by the criminal law seems preferable. The personal responsibility imposed on infected persons not to engage in behaviors reasonably likely to infect others is not disproportionate to the harm those behaviors would otherwise impose on society.

There are certain dangers in using the criminal law to discourage behavior reasonably likely to transmit HIV. Although these dangers may be kept to a minimum, they cannot be entirely eliminated. Of course, the effect of these concerns will have to be weighed against the benefit derived from the effect of such statutes in reducing HIV transmission.

One danger is that the use of the criminal law to stem HIV transmission may be counter-productive. To the extent criminal statutes directed to the prevention of HIV transmission require that a person know that he or she is infected before being subject to a criminal charge for engaging in activity likely to spread the virus, the statutes may encourage individuals to avoid testing in order to prevent establishment of a basis for subsequent criminal liability. This effect may be reduced by continued public health efforts to encourage testing, especially anonymous or confidential testing, to facilitate early access to available drug therapies that have proven most effective when instituted at an early stage of HIV infection. If testing is linked to available medical treatment rather than a need to protect others, any effect the criminal law has in discouraging testing should be minimized.

Arguably, the criminal law will have little deterrent effect on one who is HIV-infected, for that individual has already received a "death sentence" in the form of a diagnosis of HIV. For those persons whose disease has progressed from asymptomatic HIV infection to full-blown AIDS, the average survival time presently is less than two years. Hence, the threat of criminal sanction of some kind may be among the least concerns of one with AIDS.

Finally, there is a danger of selective enforcement of laws directed at HIV-transmitting activity. The possibility of arbitrary and abusive enforcement stems from the discretion such statutes place in the police and prosecuting authorities. There is a concern that such statutes may be applied selectively against gay men and other minority or unpopular groups. There is a more general concern that the public, which does not identify with these groups, may mistakenly feel that the danger of HIV infection is contained. These dangers can be avoided only by sustained public oversight of police and prosecutorial activity. The public will need to be made aware that criminal prosecution of behavior likely to result in HIV transmission does not in any way effectively remove the danger of infection to those who engage in the behaviors likely to facilitate transmission of the virus.

C. TRADITIONAL CRIMINAL OFFENSES

The designation and definition of criminal offenses varies from state to state. It therefore is necessary to examine the statutory language of the criminal code of a particular jurisdiction when attempting to determine the applicability of the criminal law to a specific act. However, it is possible to discuss traditional criminal law offenses in terms of modern statutory formulations by reference to the Model Penal Code (MPC) drafted by the American Law Institute. To a large extent, most American jurisdictions follow the MPC.

1. Murder

The MPC defines murder as the killing of another human being purposely, knowingly, or recklessly under circumstances manifesting an extreme indifference to the value of human life. MPC § 210.2. To convict an individual for murder for causing the death of another as a result of infecting the other person with HIV, the state is required to prove that the defendant knew that he or she was HIV-infected, engaged in conduct capable of transmitting HIV, and desired to cause the death of the other person, knew such conduct would cause the death of the other person, or disregarded the risk that such conduct would cause the death of another person in a way that manifests an extreme indifference to human life.

Examples of conduct engaged in with the requisite intent might include: 1) a person who deliberately causes the death of an arresting officer by stabbing the officer with a syringe containing HIV-infected fluids, 2) a prostitute who causes the death of another as a result of intercourse that the prostitute knew could lead to death because of his or her HIV infection, and, 3) a person who rapes another and causes the victim's death knowing that his or her HIV infection might have such a result.

There has not been a prosecution for murder resulting from transmission of HIV, and it is likely to be very difficult to prove murder in the case of a person who infects another with HIV. First, it would be necessary that the victim predecease the perpetrator. In most HIV transmission scenarios, the perpetrator will already be HIV-infected and thus likely to die before the victim.

Second, it would be necessary to prove that the wrongdoer was aware that he or she was HIV-positive at the time of the conduct that infected the other person. Of course, many individuals are tested anonymously at alternative test sites. Moreover, under many state laws, a person cannot be compelled to submit to AIDS-related testing or to disclose the results of such testing except under special circumstances.

Third, it would be necessary to prove that the wrongdoer knew that he or she could transfer HIV by his or her conduct and that he or she intended to infect and consequently cause the death of another person. Intentionality in the context of HIV transmission may be difficult to establish since having sex or sharing needles is a highly indirect *modus operandi* for the person whose purpose is to kill.

Fourth, it would be necessary to prove that the wrongdoer's act caused the forbidden result. In order to establish that the defendant caused the death of the victim, the prosecution must show that the defendant was HIV-infected at the time the act was committed. The prosecution also must demonstrate that the victim contracted HIV from the defendant. In order to establish the required causal connection, two negative facts must be established. First, it must be shown that the victim was not infected with HIV prior to the defendant's alleged conduct. Second, it must be proved that the victim was not infected by some other source after contact with the defendant.

A murder may someday actually be committed by transmission of HIV. In one recent robbery, the defendant threatened that the victim would get AIDS and proceeded to stab the victim with a syringe containing some kind of fluid. *State v. Caine.* There was also a case in which a prison inmate put HIV-infected blood into the coffee of a guard. *Elliott v. Dugger*.

2. Attempted Murder

A person can be convicted of attempted murder if the prosecution can prove that the individual knew or believed that he or she was HIV-infected, engaged in conduct that he or she knew or believed could transmit HIV, and did so with the purpose of causing another to become infected or did so with the belief that the behavior would produce that result.

An attempted murder charge does not require the prosecution to meet the difficult problem of proving causation presented by a charge of murder. Neither proof of the death of the victim, nor cause of death, nor actual transmission of HIV, need to be shown. However, the burden of proving the culpable state of the defendant's mind is great. In order to win a conviction for attempted murder, it must be shown that the defendant acted with the intent or purpose to cause the death of another. A person can be convicted of attempted murder if it can be shown that the person believed that his or her behavior could kill and that such a result was intended. This is true even if the wrongdoer's belief is mistaken. Thus, if an HIV-infected person spits on another person, believing that he or she can infect another person by spitting and intending to transmit HIV, he or she can be convicted of attempted murder, even if scientific and medical experts are of the opinion that HIV cannot be transmitted through spitting.

The use of an attempted murder charge to prosecute an HIV-infected offender is illustrated by *State v. Haines*. The defendant, who had attempted to commit suicide by slashing his wrists upon learning that he had AIDS, requested police and paramedics to leave him to die. When they refused his request, he began to spit, bite, scratch, and throw blood. The defendant's attempted murder conviction was affirmed on the grounds that the evidence showed the defendant was HIV-infected, was aware of his condition, believed it to be fatal, and had intended to infect others. During the struggle with the government officers, the defendant had stated his intention to infect them.

In accordance with a state statute providing that it is not a defense that, due to a misapprehension of the circumstances, it was impossible for the accused to commit the crime attempted, the court rejected the defendant's claim of impossibility. According to the court, when the defendant has done all that he or she believes necessary to cause the particular result, regardless of what is actually possible under the existing circumstances, the defendant has committed an attempt. If the defendant's conduct in light of all the reliable facts involved constitutes a substantial step toward the commission of a crime and is done with the necessary specific intent, the defendant has committed an attempt.

In another prominent attempted murder case, an HIV-infected prisoner proclaimed that he was going to infect a guard with HIV and spat in the officer's face. The prisoner's conviction for attempted murder and his life sentence were affirmed. *State v. Weeks.* Since the defendants in these types of cases are usually handcuffed, shackled, or both, they resort to spitting and biting. One might wonder whether the verbal expressions by the defendants in such cases are truly expressions of the intent to kill or are merely expressions of frustration and anger toward police and jail authorities.

In those cases in which the defendants do not verbalize their intent to transmit HIV, the difficulty in proving attempted murder is the establishment of an actual intent or motive to cause a death while believing it possible to do so by means of an HIV-infected substance. Some states have retained the defense of legal impossibility. Where this defense is available, a defendant who purposely employs some means to infect another that is incapable of transmitting HIV will be found innocent despite his or her intent. In these states, the prosecution will face an additional obstacle in cases such as those involving spitting. Most states, however, have followed the lead of the MPC and have eliminated the defense of factual impossibility. In these states, the prosecution need not prove that the conduct of the defendant actually could have caused the death of the intended victim. Rather, it need only show that the defendant did all that he or she believed was necessary to bring about the intended result of infecting another with HIV for the purpose of causing the death of the other person, regardless of the possibility of producing the intended result with the means used. *State v. Smith.*

Of course, another way to show the required intent is to prove the defendant used a deadly weapon, and the HIV virus itself has recently been held to constitute a deadly weapon where the defendant knew he was infected (and raped the victim). *Perea v. State.* In another case, where the defendant stabbed the victim with a syringe containing a clear liquid and the defendant said the victim would get AIDS, but the syringe and fluid were never found and tested for HIV, the defendant was nevertheless convicted of attempted murder. *State v. Caine.*

3. Manslaughter

Manslaughter under the MPC is a homicide that is committed by an individual with recklessness that falls short of manifesting extreme indifference to human life, but that involves a gross deviation from the standard of conduct a law abiding person would observe in a similar situation. MPC § 210.3. Recklessness involves knowledge of a substantial and unjustifiable risk that is disregarded. Whether a risk falls within the definition of a gross deviation is a question for a jury and involves weighing the risk of harm against the social utility of the conduct in which the defendant was engaged.

Knowledge of a substantial and unjustifiable risk of causing another's death might be established by showing that an individual knew that he or she was HIV-infected or was diagnosed with AIDS and also knew that the conduct in which he or she was engaged was capable of transmitting a virus that could cause death. Knowledge that one has engaged in high risk behavior and may as a result be infected might be sufficient to establish recklessness in relation to other conduct known to be capable of transmitting HIV.

A state of mind for purposes of manslaughter will be established where an actor consciously disregards a substantial and unjustifiable risk that he or she is infected. Thus, the prosecution can maintain and prove a case of manslaughter even if it cannot show that the defendant knew that he or she was infected with HIV. Nevertheless, the causation problems that exist with reference to a charge of murder also occur with the charge of manslaughter. Importantly, the victim would have to die and would have to do so before the defendant. Thus, the state would have to show that the defendant is the person from whom the decedent contracted HIV infection. Such causation is likely to be difficult to prove for the reasons described in the discussion of murder. There has not as yet been a prosecution for manslaughter resulting from transmission of HIV.

4. Negligent Homicide

Negligent homicide under the MPC occurs when an individual causes a death by engaging in conduct that the individual should be aware poses a sub-

stantial and unjustifiable risk of death to another.
MPC § 210.4. The risk must be such that it involves a gross deviation from the standard of care a
reasonable person would observe. In those jurisdictions with a statutory offense of negligent homicide,
it will be even easier to establish the culpable state
of mind than with other forms of homicide since it
is not necessary to show that a person knew of his
or her HIV condition, nor it is necessary to show
that he or she intended to infect another. Nor is it
necessary to show that the accused consciously disregarded the risk of infecting another with the
consequent risk of causing death. Rather, it is
enough to show that a defendant should have been
aware of his or her HIV infection and ability to
infect others. Again, as with other forms of homicide, the victim must die prior to the death of the
defendant in order to prosecute.

Could a person be charged with negligent homicide on the ground that he or she was a homosexual
and engaged in unprotected intercourse, even
though the person did not know that he or she was
infected or that HIV was transmitted by intercourse? Could a jury convict such a person if it
found that a reasonable person in the defendant's
circumstances would have known about their condition, known that the conduct in which they engaged
could transmit HIV, and known HIV infection is
likely to cause death, even if the defendant did not
really know any of these facts?

The principal difficulty with a charge of negligent
homicide is that of causation. It is necessary to

prove beyond a reasonable doubt that the defendant's conduct caused the victim's death. This may be difficult to establish, as suggested in the earlier discussion of causation relative to other forms of homicide. To date, there has not been a prosecution for negligent homicide resulting from transmission of HIV.

5. Assault and Battery

Assault under the MPC occurs when a person attempts to cause, or purposely, knowingly, or recklessly causes, bodily injury to another. MPC § 211.1. Many states have criminal statutes defining battery, much as with the tort distinction between assault and battery. Assault charges may be brought against an HIV-infected individual who, knowing that he or she is HIV-infected and is capable of infecting others, engages in activity likely to transmit HIV, knowing that the activity engaged in is likely to facilitate the transmission of HIV. Criminal prosecutions against HIV-infected persons under assault and battery statutes have been the most common type of AIDS-related criminal prosecution to date.

The charge of assault or battery does not require the death of the victim or even proof that the victim was infected with HIV as a result of the accused's conduct. However, consent to the conduct for which the accused is charged may be a defense. Consensual sex with an individual who informs the other person of his or her HIV infection may not involve an assault or battery. It should be noted, however, that under the MPC consent is not a defense for conduct that causes serious bodily harm. Nor does consent to sexual intercourse constitute consent to activity that might possibly lead to infection with HIV, unless the infected individual seeking consent makes full disclosure of her or his HIV status.

6. Aggravated Assault and Aggravated Battery

Aggravated assault or aggravated battery occurs when a person attempts to cause serious bodily injury to another, or causes such injury purposely, knowingly, or recklessly under circumstances that manifest extreme indifference to the value of human life. This charge can be maintained when a person attempts to cause, or purposely or knowingly causes, bodily injury to another with a deadly weapon.

An example of an HIV-related aggravated assault prosecution is provided by *United States v. Moore*. In that case, the Eighth Circuit upheld the conviction of an HIV-infected prisoner found guilty of assault with a deadly weapon for biting two prison guards during a struggle. Other courts, in non-AIDS-related prosecutions, had found use of various parts of the body to constitute a dangerous weapon, including biting with teeth and the use of fists and hands. The Eighth Circuit reasoned that assault with a dangerous weapon depends not on the nature of the object itself, but on its capacity, given the manner of its use, to endanger life or to inflict great bodily harm. Ultimately, the *Moore* court held teeth to be a dangerous weapon within the context of an aggravated assault statute regardless of the presence or absence of HIV infection in the assailant. According to the court, the record in the case, as established by expert testimony, revealed only a remote or theoretical possibility that HIV could be transmitted through biting. A similar conclusion was reached in *United States v. Sturgis*.

In another case involving an HIV-infected defendant prosecuted for biting, the Alabama Court of Criminal Appeals held that teeth do not constitute a deadly weapon within the context of an aggravated assault statute. *Brock v. State*. The defendant, who was aware that he was HIV-infected, bit two prison guards during a struggle. Although charged with attempted murder, the jury convicted the defendant of aggravated assault. On appeal, the court set aside the conviction on the ground that the record did not support the conclusion that biting could provide a source of transmission of HIV. Although the court took judicial notice of the fact that AIDS is a life-threatening disease and that contraction of HIV constitutes a serious physical injury, the court refused to take judicial notice of biting as a means capable of spreading AIDS.

7. Reckless Endangerment

Reckless endangerment under the MPC occurs when a person recklessly engages in conduct that places, or may place, another in danger of death or serious bodily injury. MPC § 211.1. It is not necessary to prove that the defendant's conduct actually harmed the other person, and consent is not a defense.

Since the mental state necessary to establish such an offense is recklessness, the jury will be required to determine whether the accused's conduct involved a gross deviation from the standard of conduct that a law abiding person would have observed in the accused's situation. When the defendant in an HIV-related prosecution is a homosexual or a drug user, there is a danger that the evaluation of the accused's conduct by a jury may be prejudiced by the accused's status.

D. RELATED CRIMINAL OFFENSES

1. Sodomy

Many states make it a crime to engage in or submit to an act of sodomy. The common law offense prohibited anal intercourse without regard to the sex or marital status of the participants. Some statutes limit their prohibitions to sexual conduct, including oral sex, between members of the same sex, while others limit their prohibitions to individuals acting outside a marital relationship. In a number of states, sodomy statutes have been found unconstitutional. In other states, the legislatures have repealed sodomy statutes or omitted a statutory provision on sodomy when enacting a new criminal code.

In *Bowers v. Hardwick*, however, the United States Supreme Court upheld a Georgia sodomy statute on the ground that such statutes do not violate the privacy protections of the federal constitution. The Court reasoned that the claim that any kind of sexual conduct between consenting adults is constitutionally insulated from state proscription is insupportable. Among the arguments made by the State of Georgia was that it was within the proper limits of the use of the police power to make acts criminal by statute that may have serious adverse consequences for the general public, such as spreading communicable diseases.

Criminally punishing sodomy in order to stem the spread of HIV infection is both an over-inclusive and under-inclusive solution. Only acts of sodomy involving an HIV-infected partner can transmit HIV. Moreover, anal intercourse with the use of a condom significantly reduces the likelihood of transmission of HIV. There is even some medical and scientific evidence that HIV cannot be transmitted by oral sex, which is included in the definition of sodomy used in many jurisdictions. Yet HIV can be transmitted by an HIV-infected partner in vaginal intercourse, which is not forbidden by any sodomy statute.

The argument that punishing sodomy is a rational means to stem HIV transmission was made in a case involving a Missouri sodomy statute specifically limited to homosexual conduct. In *State v. Walsh*, the Missouri Supreme Court upheld the statute after finding that it was rationally related to the state's legitimate interest in protecting the public health. Missouri had argued that forbidding

homosexual activity would inhibit the spread of
AIDS and other sexually communicable diseases.
The statute banned deviate sexual intercourse with
another person of the same sex and defined deviate
sexual conduct as any sexual act involving the geni-
tals of one person and the mouth, tongue, hand, or
anus of another person. The statute compounded
the problems of over- and under-inclusiveness by
forbidding mutual masturbation by same-sex partners, despite the fact that such sex has no relationship to HIV transmission. At the same time, the
statute did not forbid unprotected anal intercourse
by heterosexual partners, which is about as likely to
result in transmission of HIV as between homosexual partners.

2. Prostitution

Prostitution is a crime in every state except Nevada, where each county has the option of criminalizing or licensing the activity. The traditional definition of prostitution includes the practice of a female
offering her body for indiscriminate intercourse for
money or hire. Modern statutes have been expanded to include male prostitutes, including those engaging in homosexual acts. The MPC applies to a
person who engages in sexual activity as a business
and includes homosexual and deviate sexual relations within the definition of sexual activity. MPC
§ 251.2.

Where an HIV-infected person is engaged in prostitution and is performing sexual acts likely to
transmit HIV, existing laws punishing prostitution

may be appropriately invoked to stem HIV transmission. Such prosecutions have resulted in some cases in the isolation through house arrest of HIV-infected prostitutes. Similarly, where a state has a law prohibiting patronizing a prostitute, infected patrons of prostitutes can be prosecuted and sentenced.

Some states have developed specific offenses, such as aggravated prostitution, aimed at prostitutes who know they are HIV-positive and continue to engage in sexual conduct likely to transmit HIV. Florida law, for example, provides for the prosecution of any person committing prostitution after testing positive for HIV knowing that he or she can transmit the virus to others. The sexual activity must be of the type likely to transmit the virus. The statute also provides that a person may be convicted and sentenced separately for the HIV-specific offense and for the underlying crime of prostitution. Florida law also provides for the conviction of an HIV-infected person procuring another to commit prostitution in a manner likely to transmit HIV when the person has tested positive for HIV and knows or has been informed of his or her infection.

3. Rape

According to the MPC, rape occurs when a male has sexual intercourse with a female, not his wife, as a result of compelling her to submit by force, threat of serious bodily injury, extreme pain, or kidnapping. MPC § 213.1. Some states, such as

Illinois, have designated this offense "criminal sexual assault" and provide for the charge of aggravated criminal sexual assault when an accused causes bodily harm to a victim. At a minimum, transmission of HIV during rape is a factor in aggravation. *People v. Johnson*.

For rape to exist, sexual intercourse must occur by force or intimidation. The force of intercourse itself will establish the *actus reus* of the offense if sexual intercourse occurs without the woman's consent. If consent was obtained without the male disclosing that he was HIV-infected, or if the male falsely denied HIV infection, the question arises whether such consent is effective to constitute a defense. Generally, actual consent, even if obtained by fraud, is an affirmative defense to a charge of rape. *United States v. Booker*.

Certain states, such as Florida, now permit rape victims to demand that their attackers undergo HIV testing for the purpose of determining whether the victim is at risk of developing AIDS due to the rape.

4. Use of Controlled Substances

Sharing needles in illicit intravenous drug use is a primary means of transmitting HIV. There are both federal and state laws directed at unlawful drug sale, possession, and use. Some states have statutes prohibiting the possession of instruments adapted for use of controlled substances or the exchange or sale of such instruments.

It has been argued that vigorous enforcement of laws related to controlled substances and those prohibiting the sale or exchange of needles may reduce transmission of HIV by discouraging intravenous drug use. Others argue that the enforcement of laws related to the possession and sale of needles may increase the transmission of HIV by increasing the sharing of dirty needles.

E. PUBLIC HEALTH OFFENSES

1. Transmission of Communicable Diseases

A number of states have statutes that make it a criminal offense for a person with a contagious disease to willfully or knowingly transmit to or expose another person to that disease. These statutes provide criminal penalties for public health offenses that are otherwise dealt with by civil quarantine or isolation.

Some of these statutes have special elements, such as requiring that the conduct occur in a public place. Most treat willful communication of or exposure to a communicable disease as a misdemeanor punishable by fines or by imprisonment for no more than a year. Some of these statutes define communicable disease by reference to specified diseases. Some states have explicitly amended their statutes to include intentional exposure to HIV.

2. Sexually Transmitted Diseases

Many states have provisions specifically criminalizing willful or knowing exposure of another to a

sexually transmitted disease. Typically, these statutes impose a criminal penalty for the transmission
of a communicable venereal disease through sexual
intercourse, but some states make it a crime to
willfully "expose" another person to a venereal
disease. Courts have long upheld imposition of
prison sentences for violation of these statutes.

Many jurisdictions have not yet included HIV
infection as a designated venereal disease. However, some states have added HIV infection or AIDS
to the enumeration of venereal diseases. In certain
states, a designated authority, such as the commissioner of health, has authority to promulgate a list
of sexually transmitted diseases. Some jurisdictions include broad language, such as "any other
disease which can be sexually transmitted," and
such language undoubtedly could be construed to
include HIV infection.

Many of these statutes grade such offenses as a
misdemeanor. Some states impose broad bans that
prohibit infected persons from engaging in sexual
intercourse. Such prohibitions raise serious questions of appropriateness when dealing with HIV,
particularly since safe sexual practices between
partners can virtually eliminate the risk of transmission.

F. HIV–SPECIFIC OFFENSES

In response to the perceived inadequacies of the
traditional criminal law in punishing and deterring
conduct by HIV-infected persons likely to result in

transmission of HIV, a number of state legislatures have enacted or proposed legislation making it a criminal offense for an HIV-infected person to knowingly engage in activity likely to result in the transmission of HIV.

The Presidential Commission on the Human Immunodeficiency Virus Epidemic observed in its final report that problems in applying traditional criminal law to HIV transmission should lead to the adoption of criminal statutes specific to HIV infection. According to the Commission, an HIV-specific statute can provide clear notice of socially unacceptable standards of behavior specific to the HIV epidemic and can facilitate tailoring punishment to the specific crime of HIV-transmitting behavior.

While the enacted and proposed HIV-specific laws have varied from state to state, such statutes uniformly make it an offense for an HIV-infected person to knowingly engage in behavior likely to transmit HIV. Some of the statutes avoid the problems created by the more traditional offenses, which require proof of intent, purpose, causation, or actual injury. The majority of the statutes have classified the proscribed behavior as a felony, thus avoiding the criticism leveled at other offenses available for prosecuting HIV-transmitting activity, such as reckless endangerment, as being too lenient where the transmitting activity is engaged in knowingly or intentionally. The advantage of HIV-specific criminal laws is that they are, for the most part, narrowly drafted to address particular conduct that places others at risk of infection with HIV.

The laws that have been proposed or enacted thus far have been directed either to conduct that is specially designated, such as donation of blood by a person who knows that he or she is HIV-infected, or to more general conduct likely to transmit HIV by a person who knows that he or she is HIV-infected.

HIV-specific criminal offenses convey the most effective warning and have the maximum deterrent value. These statutes can identify the specific conduct necessary to avoid or reduce the likelihood of HIV infection. There is, however, some difficulty on the part of legislatures in explaining exactly what is prohibited. For instance, the Illinois statute describes the conduct forbidden by the term "intimate conduct" as "exposure of the body of one person to a bodily fluid of another person in a manner that could result in transmission of HIV." This language fails to achieve the specificity necessary to describe the conduct forbidden and will require judicial construction. A more effective approach is taken by the Michigan statute, which uses the term "sexual penetration" and defines it as "sexual intercourse, cunnilingus, fellatio, anal intercourse, or any other intrusion, however slight, of any part of a person's body or of any object into the genital or anal openings of another person's body, but emission of semen is not required."

One type of HIV-specific criminal statute is aimed at preventing transmission of HIV through donation of infected blood or blood products. For example, Indiana imposes penalties on persons who recklessly or knowingly donate blood, blood components, or semen knowing that they are HIV-infected or that they have tested positive for the antibody to HIV. This statute avoids the problems of proof required by traditional criminal offenses. For the basic offense, no causation needs to be established. Moreover, the statute does not require proof that the defendant intended to infect others. Rather, it is enough for the prosecution to show that a donor was reckless with regard to whether donated blood or semen was HIV-infected. Of course, where it can be shown that the donor knew that HIV-infected material was being transferred or intended to transfer such material, liability is easily established.

Some states have enacted statutes that impose criminal penalties on persons who engage in sexual conduct, often specified as sexual intercourse or penetration, knowing they have tested HIV-positive or have been diagnosed with AIDS. Some of these laws specifically recognize a defense of consent or make such sexual conduct a crime only if the actor's sexual partner has not been notified of the actor's condition. The Michigan act is a typical example of this type of statute. The law provides in part: "A person who knows that he or she has or has been diagnosed as having acquired immunodeficiency syndrome or acquired immunodeficiency syndrome-related complex, or who knows that he or she is HIV-infected, and who engages in sexual penetration with another person without having first informed the other person that he or she has acquired immunodeficiency syndrome or acquired immunodeficiency syndrome-related complex or is HIV-infected, is guilty of a felony.''

Some states have imposed enhanced penalties on persons who commit a sex offense or engage in prostitution knowing that they are HIV-infected. The Florida statute establishes the crime of engaging in prostitution while HIV-infected. The statute provides that a person may be convicted separately for a violation of this statute as well as for the underlying crime of prostitution. The Florida statute specifies that the sexual activity at issue must be of the type likely to transmit HIV to others.

One state, Oklahoma, enacted a statute criminalizing any conduct by an HIV-infected person that is likely to transmit HIV. The problem with this type of statute is that the lack of specification of forbidden conduct creates the need for considerable judicial construction in order to avoid problems of vagueness and lack of notice. Another problem is that this type of statute continues the requirement of proof of intentionality that results in the traditional offenses being of limited use in dealing with activity likely to transmit HIV.

To date, there have been only a few challenges to the constitutionality of HIV-specific criminal statutes. In each instance, the law has been upheld as applied to the particular circumstances of the case involved. *People v. Russell.*

G. DEFENSES

1. Consent

Under the MPC, consent of the victim is a defense only when it negates an element of the offense or precludes the infliction of the harm or evil sought to be prevented by the law defining the offense. MPC § 2.11(1). When serious bodily harm will result from the conduct, consent will not be a defense. In the case of conduct likely to transmit HIV, because the effect of infection is serious injury and likely death, consent will not be available as a defense to a traditional criminal offense such as murder. However, consent is available as a defense when the statutory formulation expressly recognizes it as an affirmative defense. The Illinois statute on criminal transmission of HIV, for example, specifically provides for such an affirmative defense. In a court martial proceeding, however, a military tribunal refused to recognize consent to sex with a soldier known to have HIV as a defense, due to the overriding societal interest in preventing the spread of AIDS. *United States v. Morris.*

2. Mistake

Ignorance or mistake of fact or law under the MPC is a defense when it negates the existence of a mental state essential to the crime charged. MPC § 2.04(1)(a). This defense prevents conviction when it is shown that the defendant did not have the mental state required by law for the commission of the particular offense. For instance, the Michigan statute provides for the offense of engaging in sexual penetration when an individual knows that he or she is HIV-infected. If the person is unaware of his or her HIV status or is mistaken as to whether he or she is infected, there would seem to be a defense to a charge under the Michigan statute. Perhaps if the infected individual insisted on the use of a condom, in the mistaken belief that it is 100% effective in preventing the transmission of HIV, he or she might have a defense. It has been held, however, that the use of a condom in a case involving sexual penetration does not negate criminal intent. *United States v. Joseph.*

3. Impossibility

The defense of legal impossibility provides a defense and is available when what the defendant sets out to do is not criminal. Factual impossibility, which normally does not provide a defense, occurs when defendants are unable to accomplish what they intend because of some fact that is unknown to them. In the HIV context, legal impossibility would occur, for instance, if an HIV-infected person were to believe that he or she had committed a crime by not informing one's barber or hairstylist of his or her HIV status when, in fact, there is no law requiring such disclosure. Factual impossibility would occur if an HIV-infected person intended to kill another by spitting on the victim, even though expert medical testimony establishes that it is not possible to transmit HIV by such means. But the use of a condom in the case of alleged sexual exposure to HIV would not constitute legal or factual impossibility. *United States v. Joseph.*

The modern view is that impossibility is not a defense when the defendant's actual intent is to do an act or bring about a result proscribed by law. The MPC provides that a person is guilty of a crime if he or she "purposely engages in conduct which would constitute a crime if the attendant circumstances were as he [or she] believes them to be." MPC § 5.01(1)(a). This approach is illustrated by the case of *State v. Haines.* A person infected with HIV announced that he had AIDS and that he was going to show everyone what it was like to have the disease. He then began to spit, bite, scratch, and throw blood on his intended victims. The Indiana Court of Appeals upheld an attempted murder conviction on the ground that it is no defense to a charge of attempt that because of a misapprehension of the circumstances, it was impossible for the accused to commit the crime attempted.

H. MANDATORY HIV TESTING

There have been numerous legislative efforts to enact mandatory HIV testing provisions in connection with a variety of criminal offenses. Not surprisingly, this has proven to be a very complicated and controversial matter. Should one who has merely been arrested for an enumerated offense be subjected to mandatory testing, or should such testing be limited to individuals who have been convicted? Which offenses should trigger such testing?

Where a sex offense is involved, should the victim be informed of the results of the defendant's HIV test? Should any special provisions be applied where the offender or the victim is a juvenile?

Statutes have been adopted authorizing mandatory HIV testing for those convicted, and sometimes even simply arrested, for certain sex offenses and drug offenses. Often the victim is entitled to be informed of the test results of the offender (or alleged offender).

These mandatory HIV testing laws are subject to attack on a variety of state and federal constitutional grounds. Although there have not yet been many such challenges, at least one trial court has struck down one mandatory testing statute as unconstitutional. *In re J.G.*

I. SENTENCING

Should the fact of a defendant's HIV infection constitute either an aggravating or a mitigating factor at the sentencing stage of the proceedings? Or is HIV infection irrelevant? It depends. Certainly, if HIV infection is an element of the crime involved, the HIV infection of the defendant will be known to the court at sentencing. Judges have displayed a range of views about HIV.

Some judges have shown great compassion for those with HIV and have imposed light prison sentences, even sentencing some offenders to mere probation (if HIV is unrelated to the crime and if the crime was not a violent one). Occasionally, at-home detention of HIV-infected individuals has been imposed, particularly where short jail terms otherwise would have been involved and where some sort of electronic monitoring is available.

On the other hand, some judges have sentenced HIV-infected defendants to long prison terms, apparently to keep these infected individuals segregated from the general public for as long as possible. Of course, it is well known that an HIV diagnosis is effectively a "death sentence" for the infected individual and that a prison term of even modest length can effectively be a "life sentence" for such a person.

The question of what role AIDS should play in sentencing (as well as early release) decisions has recently been brought into sharp focus. In *United States v. Streat*, a federal district court in Ohio held that AIDS can be taken into account during sentencing. Just a short time later, however, the Eighth Circuit concluded that AIDS does not authorize a downward departure from the federal sentencing guidelines. *United States v. Rabins*. As the number of prisoners with AIDS grows, this issue is certain to be faced by many more courts.

CHAPTER VI

TORT LAW

A. INTRODUCTION

The primary focus in litigation involving tort liability related to AIDS has involved suits arising from breach of duty resulting in transmission of HIV. Tort law is a legal mechanism used to discourage individuals from subjecting others to unreasonable risks and to compensate those who have been injured by unreasonably risky behavior. The greatest number of AIDS-related liability lawsuits have alleged the receipt of HIV-infected blood and blood products. There also have been a number of suits filed relating to the sexual transmission of HIV. A third area of litigation that has been spawned by AIDS involves suits for AIDS-related psychic distress. Patients have sought damages for emotional duress upon learning that they have been treated by HIV-infected physicians who have performed exposure-prone procedures on these patients.

B. BLOOD AND BLOOD PRODUCTS

The question of liability for supplying HIV-infected blood or plasma prior to the development of the antibody test is a complex matter. By the end of

176

1982, evidence had developed that AIDS was associated with blood transfusions and with the antihemophilic factor. As a result of studies carried out by the PHS, general recommendations for preventing transmission of AIDS through blood and blood products were developed. These recommendations resulted in the issuance of specific guidelines by the FDA in 1983 to all blood- and plasma-collecting facilities in the United States. The guidelines called for collection centers to provide information about AIDS to donors so that they would be able to determine if they were members of groups at increased risks. The guidelines also suggested revising standard operating procedures to include specific questions regarding signs and symptoms of AIDS and advising donors that those at increased risk of AIDS should voluntarily decline to give blood.

In addition to the FDA, the CDC also studied the problem of blood donations. It was decided that since no specific test was known to detect AIDS at an early stage in a potential donor, all members of groups at increased risk for AIDS should refrain from donating. Government and industry representatives concluded that no other viable alternative existed in the absence of a reliable screening mechanism.

1. Negligence and Standard of Care

Transmission of AIDS through blood products, including cases involving transfusions and the providing of the plasma blood product Factor–VIII to hemophiliacs, has been a major area of litigation activity. A claim of liability against a hospital or blood bank that provides infected blood is most usually based on the contention that the hospital or blood bank negligently supplied unfit blood for patient use.

There has been considerable litigation on the issue of what standard of care should apply in negligence cases involving the transfusion of HIV-contaminated blood before the development of HIV antibody testing. In these cases, the plaintiffs typically allege that the defendants were negligent in failing to implement safety measures, such as donor screening, surrogate testing, heat treatment, or autologous or directed donations.

Several courts have ruled that defendants cannot be held liable for negligence for supplying or transfusing HIV-contaminated blood if they adhered to industry-wide custom. For example, in *Seitzinger v. American Red Cross*, a Pennsylvania federal court dismissed a negligence claim against a blood bank. The court held that as a matter of law, the blood bank could not be found negligent because it had followed prevailing industry customs, which in 1983 did not include heat treatment or surrogate testing.

Several courts, however, have been unwilling to summarily dispose of negligence claims. Instead, they have required a factual determination of the state of medical knowledge at the time of the fateful transfusion and the defendant's level of awareness about the possibility of transmitting HIV by blood or blood products.

In *United Blood Services v. Quintana*, the plaintiff received a blood transfusion during surgery in 1983. She developed AIDS and died in 1985. At trial, the plaintiff claimed that the supplier of the HIV-contaminated blood was negligent for failing to question donors about risk factors for HIV infection and for failing to implement surrogate testing. The defendant asserted that it was not negligent because its blood testing procedures conformed with industry custom and FDA regulations. The jury returned a verdict for the defendant, which was affirmed on appeal.

The Colorado Supreme Court, however, reversed and remanded the case for another trial, holding that adherence to the prevailing standard of care among blood banks was not conclusive proof of the exercise of due care. The court found that the trial judge had erred in excluding evidence that the defendant should have known in 1983 that HIV was blood-borne and, as a consequence, that its safety procedures were "unreasonably deficient." The court explained that:

> [A] plaintiff should be permitted to present expert opinion testimony that the standard of care adopted by the school of practice to which the defendant adheres is unreasonably deficient by not incorporating readily available practices and procedures substantially more protective against the harm caused to the plaintiff than the stan-

dard of care adopted by the defendant's school of practice.

After the new trial, the jury awarded $8.1 million to the plaintiff.

2. Screening Tests

The availability since 1985 of the HIV antibody test has permitted organizations that collect blood and plasma to screen donations for HIV antibodies in accordance with guidelines developed by the CDC. Under the guidelines, blood or plasma that is positive on initial testing cannot be transfused or manufactured into other products capable of transmitting infectious agents. Since the proportion of false positive results is high, the incidence of false negatives is low, and the prevalence of HIV infection in the general population is small, the antibody test is highly effective in detecting infected blood. In order to minimize the number of false negative test results, it has been further recommended that members of groups at increased risk for AIDS refrain from donating blood and plasma.

It should be recognized that some risk still remains due to the fact that blood that produces a negative reaction to the test may carry the virus. Studies have reported several cases in which the antibody has not been detected in asymptomatic individuals infected with HIV for more than six months. Since blood from such persons will not produce a positive antibody test result, physicians and providers administering blood and blood products should inform the prospective recipient of the continuing risk of infection from these products. Such informed consent may preclude liability on the part of a physician or health care provider absent a showing of negligence in the use of the screening procedures.

3. Autologous and Directed Donations

Because of the small but identifiable risk of HIV infection to recipients of screened blood, those providing blood should consider making available to recipients autologous and directed donations. An autologous donation involves taking blood from an individual for future use by the patient. This procedure is highly recommended where a patient is undergoing elective surgery. Another measure that may be offered is that of directed donation, by which specially identified individuals donate blood for the use of an identified patient. It is arguable that this provides no real assurance of HIV-free blood. Nevertheless, several states, such as California, require that patients be advised of the availability of directed donations.

4. Breach of Implied Warranty

An action for breach of an implied warranty is based on statutes that establish contractual warranties for the sale of products. In the case of a sale of blood, the seller is bound by an implied warranty that the blood and blood products sold to the patient are fit for transfusion.

In deciding HIV transfusion liability, most courts considering the matter have held that hospitals supplying blood are not liable for breaches of implied warranties. They have done so on the basis that blood transfusions constitute a service rather than the sale of a product. *Perlmutter v. Beth David Hospital*. However, in *Doe v. Miles Laboratories, Inc.*, a Maryland federal court found that blood supplied by a blood bank is a product and, as such, is subject to an implied warranty of fitness. Nevertheless, most states have adopted statutes shielding blood suppliers from liability by providing, as a matter of state law, that the procurement and supplying of blood is to be treated as a service and not as a sale of a commodity, thus precluding a claim for damages based on any implied warranty.

5. Strict Liability in Tort

A possible basis for an action against a hospital or blood bank supplying HIV-infected blood might be strict liability in tort. In *Cunningham v. MacNeal Memorial Hospital*, the Illinois Supreme Court ruled that a hospital could be held strictly liable for supplying hepatitis-contaminated blood to a patient. The court explicitly rejected a loophole for "unavoidably unsafe products" that provides an exception from strict liability for a product that cannot be made fully safe for its intended use given the current state of scientific knowledge. The court ruled that this exception was intended to apply to "pure" but sometimes unsafe products, such as the vaccine for rabies, but was not meant to apply to "impure" substances such as blood containing the hepatitis B virus.

Most states have now adopted statutes that eliminate liability without fault for those who dispense blood products. These statutes declare blood transfusions to be a service exempt from the rule of strict liability for a defective product. In those states that have not adopted such statutes, the general rule appears to be that suppliers of blood containing HIV may rely on the "unavoidably unsafe products" exception to the rule of strict liability where there is no known mechanism to ascertain that blood is contaminated by a virus. While this rule provides a defense to liability for blood supplied before the development of the HIV antibody tests, protection from liability after the test became available requires that all blood supplies be screened for the antibody.

As noted above, most states confer some form of statutory immunity from implied warranties and strict liability for suppliers of blood and blood products. It is necessary to examine the statute of each jurisdiction to determine the coverage of the statute. Such statutes vary in coverage and may or may not include one or more of the following entities: hospitals, blood banks, for-profit collectors, processors, and distributors. Statutes also differ in the material covered. While some refer only to whole blood, others include plasma, blood products, blood components, and blood derivatives. Statutes also vary in the transmitted diseases covered. Some statutes specify illnesses such as hepatitis. Others include HIV or AIDS. Some statutes bar strict liability, but make no reference to implied warranties. Others, such as the California statute, declare that everything having to do with blood is a service and not a sale, thus barring both strict liability and implied warranties.

6. Informed Consent and Negligent Representation

The duty to avoid negligence may include obtaining informed consent from the patient before administering a transfusion or providing other blood products. This is especially true in relation to HIV testing because of the possibility of a false negative result due to the extended incubation period of the virus. Moreover, if blood has been obtained from paid donors, the patient should be informed of the increased risks faced by accepting such blood. Some states have enacted statutes requiring that blood obtained from paid donors be labeled to indicate this fact. Informed consent will not provide a defense in a suit for negligence because such consent is effective only if the blood supplier has done all that is reasonably possible to ensure that the blood is free from HIV infection.

7. Discovery

The issue of discovery of information about donors has arisen in suits against blood banks and hospitals that have distributed HIV-contaminated blood and in suits against suppliers of blood products that allegedly resulted in transmission of HIV. Blood banks and hospitals have opposed the disclosure of the identities of blood donors on the grounds that they have an obligation to protect donor privacy and that the public interest in encouraging blood donation would be frustrated if there was a possibility that a donor's identity could be revealed.

Courts have split on the issue of protecting donor identities. The majority position is to protect donor identities in civil cases. The principal arguments against discovery have been that blood donor identities fall within the scope of the physician-patient privilege, that such identities are protected under a constitutional right of privacy, and that the identities of donors are protected by abuse-of-discovery rules under which the court must prohibit discovery that will cause unreasonable expense or intrusion. Courts that have applied such abuse-of-discovery rules have concluded that injury to the public's interest in an adequate volunteer blood supply weighs in favor of prohibiting discovery of donor identities.

8. Treatment by an HIV–Infected Physician

A few courts have recognized claims of patients based on fear of contracting AIDS from an HIV-infected physician. For example, in *Faya v. Almaraz*, the Maryland Supreme Court upheld a claim of AIDS-phobia by two patients who sued their former physician after they learned that he had been HIV-positive when he had performed surgery on them. The court held that the plaintiffs were not required to prove that they were actually exposed to HIV.

Instead, they only needed to establish that their fear was reasonable.

By contrast, California courts have required plaintiffs to satisfy the "more likely than not" standard, first adopted in cancer-phobia cases, in order to recover emotional distress claims arising out of negligent exposure to HIV or AIDS. Absent proof of present physical injury or illness, this standard requires the plaintiff to show he or she will more likely than not develop the feared HIV or AIDS in the future due to the alleged exposure.

C. SEXUAL TRANSMISSION

1. Negligence

Liability for negligence for sexual transmission of AIDS requires establishing a duty on the part of the person transmitting AIDS that arises from the relationship between the sexual partners, a breach of that duty, a causal relationship between the defendant's conduct and the injury suffered by the sexual partner, and damages or loss to the plaintiff.

It is easily foreseeable that a person who knows that he or she is infected with HIV or has contracted AIDS may infect a sexual partner with the virus with a resultant development of AIDS, thereby giving rise to a duty to disclose the existence of infection to partners. Even those courts that hesitate to find such a broad general duty might find a duty in the nature of the relationship existing between the parties. In the landmark case of *Crowell v. Crowell*, a woman successfully sued her husband for wrongfully and recklessly infecting her with a "loathsome disease." In finding that the defendant had breached his duty, the North Carolina Supreme Court relied heavily on the marital relationship between the sexual partners. Subsequent cases have found that an intimate sexual relationship itself gives rise to a duty. The result is that the rules of negligence are equally applicable whether or not the persons involved are married to each other.

Courts will impose a duty of care if a defendant had actual knowledge of his or her HIV infection. Courts appear unwilling, however, to impose a duty upon defendants merely because they have been sexually active. In *Doe v. Johnson*, for example, the court rejected the plaintiff's argument that basketball star Magic Johnson had a duty to warn her that he might be HIV-positive before they had sex merely because he had led a "promiscuous, sexually active and multiple partner" lifestyle. Instead, the court held that such a duty arises only if a defendant has actual knowledge of his or her serostatus, has experienced HIV-related symptoms, or has actual knowledge that a former sexual partner has been diagnosed as HIV positive.

However, in *Meany v. Meany*, the Supreme Court of Louisiana held that because the defendant-husband had engaged in multiple extramarital sexual affairs for which he could not testify with certainty that protective devices were used, and because he had sought medical attention for "drippage," he had a duty to either refrain from sexual contact with his wife or to warn her of his symptoms. The fact that he did not know that he was infected with herpes was deemed irrelevant, as was the fact that drippage is not a symptom normally associated with herpes. The court reasoned that the defendant's sexual promiscuity and drippage problem were enough to show that the defendant knew, or should have suspected, that he was putting his wife at risk of venereal disease.

2. Battery

A battery is an intentional and unprivileged contact with the person of another that is harmful or offensive. To establish a battery, it ordinarily is necessary to show that the defendant intended to cause an unprivileged contact. In the case of AIDS, the unprivileged contact normally will be the transmission of the virus, although it may be enough to show that the defendant knew that he or she was infected with HIV or had contracted AIDS and intended to cause the sexual contact that in turn caused transmission of the virus. In a landmark case, *State v. Lankford*, the Delaware Supreme Court upheld a husband's conviction of criminal assault and battery for transmitting syphilis to his wife. The court determined that the element of intent was established when it was shown that the husband had intercourse knowing that he had contracted syphilis. Although that case involved a criminal prosecution for battery, the elements of civil and criminal battery are essentially the same. In contrast to a suit for negligence, in which it may be enough to show that a tortfeasor should have known of his or her infected condition, a battery claim requires a showing that the person transmitting the disease had actual knowledge of his or her infected condition.

3. Misrepresentation

An actionable misrepresentation is established by showing that the plaintiff reasonably relied, to his or her detriment, on the defendant's knowing or negligent misrepresentation of a material fact. To establish fraud in a case of transmission of HIV or for contracting AIDS, a plaintiff must show that the defendant actually knew of his or her infectious condition and withheld that information with the purpose of inducing the plaintiff to have sex.

Mark Christian, the gay lover of Rock Hudson, was awarded $21.75 million by a California jury in 1989. Christian argued that Hudson had concealed his HIV seropositivity from Christian throughout much of their relationship, and that he had consented to sexual activity without using barrier contraceptives in ignorance of Hudson's HIV infection. Christian claimed that he had first learned of Hudson's condition when it became public knowledge shortly before Hudson's death in 1985. Christian continued to test HIV-negative at the time of the trial, years after Hudson's death.

4. Liability Based on Statutory Violation

Many states have enacted statutes making the communication of venereal disease a crime. Typically, these statutes impose a criminal penalty for the transmission of a communicable venereal disease through sexual intercourse, although some states make it a crime to wilfully "expose" another person to a venereal disease. Courts have upheld convictions and the imposition of prison sentences for violations of these statutes, and some have gone further and authorized a private right of action for money damages as a result of the plaintiff having contracted a sexually transmitted disease. Where negligence *per se* is recognized, a defendant's claim that he or she exercised due care generally will not result in an escape from liability. A minority of courts, however, find a violation of such a statute to be only evidence of negligence.

The primary obstacle to basing tort liability on a statute that provides criminal penalties for communicating a venereal disease is that in many jurisdictions AIDS is not yet officially recognized as a venereal disease. However, some jurisdictions include broad language such as "any other disease which can be sexually transmitted," and such language undoubtedly can be construed to include AIDS.

5. Defenses

Each of the various causes of action that potentially offer a basis for a civil suit by a person who has been infected with HIV, or who has developed AIDS as a result of transmission of the virus by another individual, is subject to one or more defenses. Assumption of risk and contributory negligence may provide defenses in suits based on negligence; consent may be offered as a defense in an action for battery. Interspousal immunity, illegality of the underlying conduct, and the right of privacy of a sexual partner also provide potential obstacles to recovery in tort actions for damages for the sexual transmission of HIV.

a. Assumption of Risk

When a person infected with HIV or diagnosed as having AIDS accurately informs a prospective sexual partner of his or her condition and the partner understands the risk and voluntarily consents to sexual activity, the partner has expressly assumed the risk of contracting AIDS. Thus, no liability will ensue for its transmission.

The question arises whether a person who consents to sexual relations implicitly assumes the risk of contracting AIDS, given the widespread knowledge of the nature of the disease and the means of transmission. This defense is not likely to prevail, however, because assumption of risk involves a subjective standard and courts are unwilling to require that common knowledge be included in any given person's actual knowledge.

In general, since the state has an interest in the health and welfare of all its citizens, particularly in the area of the transmission of a venereal or contagious disease, it seems unlikely that a court would recognize a defense based on an implied assumption of the risk that one might contract AIDS from sexual relations.

b. Contributory Negligence

Since a reasonable person would realize that his or her non-monogamous sexual relationships significantly increase the chances of contracting AIDS, promiscuity might be considered contributory negligence. Contributory negligence also might lie in the failure to wear a condom or to ask a partner to wear one. Generally engaging in unsafe sexual practices also may count as contributory negligence.

In a comparative negligence state, a plaintiff's damages will be decreased by the amount that his or her negligence contributed to contracting the disease.

c. Interspousal Immunity

In recent years, the doctrine of interspousal immunity has been increasingly rejected. The contemporary position is that neither spouse is immune from tort liability to the other solely by reason of the marital relationship. In those states that have abrogated the doctrine, suits for battery for transmission of HIV or AIDS will not be barred. In states that have rejected interspousal immunity only in cases of intentional torts, a spouse would have to sue for battery rather than negligence in order to recover for transmission of HIV or for contracting AIDS from a spouse. Some states allow such action only after the marriage has been terminated by divorce.

Courts in states that adhere to the doctrine of spousal immunity have held that it does not apply to torts committed before the marriage. In such a jurisdiction, persons who could show that they had been exposed to the virus or contracted the disease from sexual activities with their spouse before they were married will be able to sue their spouse for transmitting a disease.

d. Illegality

Where AIDS is transmitted as a result of sexual activity between unmarried persons, the defendant may be able to raise the defense of illegality. In many jurisdictions the underlying sexual activity will violate statutory prohibitions against fornication, sodomy, or adultery. However, the defense of illegality in the context of sexual relations has eroded over the years. Some courts that continue to recognize that defense have limited it to situations where the parties are of equal guilt.

In *Neal v. Neal*, the Idaho Supreme Court denied a wife tort recovery for damages for the adulterous relationship of her husband based on theories of criminal conversation, invasion of privacy, interference with contract, and violation of the statutory duty of fiduciary.

Courts have been increasingly willing to provide recovery where a partner causes injury or knowingly transmits an incurable disease to an innocent party as a result of sexual relations, regardless of the partners' marital status. However, in the *Neal* case, the court denied the wife recovery for emotional distress from fear of contracting a sexually transmitted disease from her adulterous husband.

e. Right to Privacy

An action seeking judicial imposition of tort liability for sexual transmission of HIV or AIDS must overcome the assertion that it violates the constitutional right to privacy. Courts have been reluctant to sanction state intrusion into private relationships. The question arises, however, whether such intrusion is warranted under particular circumstances.

In *Kathleen K. v. Robert B.*, the California Court of Appeals reasoned that the constitutional right to privacy does not preclude an unmarried woman from suing a man in tort for transmitting herpes to her through sexual intercourse. The defendant maintained that it was not the business of the judiciary to supervise the promises or claims made between two consenting adults concerning the circumstances of their private sexual conduct. The court responded to this argument by stating that the right of privacy is not absolute, and in some instances must be subordinated to the state's fundamental right to enact laws promoting the public health and the welfare and safety of its citizens.

D. DRUG USE

Nonmedical drugs are often injected by persons sharing needles without cleaning or sterilizing the needles between uses. This practice enables blood containing contaminants such as HIV to pass from person to person. The transmission of AIDS among intravenous drug users is thought to occur as a result of sharing or reusing blood-contaminated needles and syringes in "shooting galleries," the apartments and other locations in metropolitan areas that are frequented by drug users.

1. Battery

A person who intentionally or knowingly induces another person to use a needle contaminated with HIV commits a battery, which is an intentional, harmful, or offensive unprivileged contact with the person of another. A defendant's liability for battery extends to consequences that the defendant did not intend and could not reasonably foresee. Thus, a defendant who knowingly causes another person to be infected with HIV could be liable if the other person developed AIDS; in fact, the defendant may be liable in battery merely for transmitting HIV. Where a battery is established, the defendant may be liable not only to the person who becomes infected with HIV, or to his or her survivor in a wrongful death suit, but also to any offspring who becomes infected.

2. Negligence

Needle-sharers have a legal duty not to infect each other. A prudent person could clearly foresee that a shared needle can transmit HIV. The burden of guarding against that event is not great. One can either not share needles or else sterilize them before reuse. Finally, the burden of avoiding needle-carried HIV infection imposes little hardship on the persons involved and is of great social benefit in reducing the incidence of AIDS.

With the existence and scope of duty established, one would next need to establish a breach of duty to show that the defendant's conduct fell below the standard of care required. Given the general understanding of the danger of transmitting HIV, a person inducing another to share unclean needles clearly fails to meet the standard of conduct of a reasonable and prudent person.

The plaintiff, of course, must establish that his or her injuries were caused by the defendant's breach of some duty that was owed to the plaintiff. A factor cited frequently by courts in determining the existence and scope of a duty is the foreseeability of the possible harm. Additional factors that may be taken into account in establishing the existence and scope of a legal duty include the likelihood of injury, the magnitude of the burden of guarding against the injury, and the consequences of placing the burden of the duty on the defendant. One may establish a duty on the part of a person inducing another to share needles or by sharing the needles of another knowing of the likelihood of the transmission of HIV by showing that it is clearly foreseeable to a prudent person that sharing needles may result in transmission of the virus.

3. Causation

In order to recover damages on the basis of negligence in the transmission of HIV or in contracting AIDS through the use of shared needles, a plaintiff must show that a particular incident in which needles were shared was the cause of the transmission of the virus. As a practical matter, given the fact that it is not likely that such conduct will involve an isolated instance of sharing needles, proof of causation may pose an insurmountable difficulty. However, if one could show that transmission occurred through an isolated instance of sharing needles and that no other activity could have made transmission possible, one may be able to establish the necessary causal relationship between transmission and the negligence of the person inducing the sharing of needles.

4. Consent and Illegality

Because the intravenous drug use related to HIV transmission generally involves a violation of the criminal law, the plaintiff's consensual participation in that criminal activity may affect the defendant's liability. Nevertheless, conduct committed with the intention of inflicting harm on another is ordinarily a crime despite the fact that the party harmed has consented to the conduct causing the harm. A number of courts similarly have held that consent will not protect a defendant against civil liability for damages in cases of mutual physical combat and battery.

The strongest case for disallowing consent as a defense to a tort claim is where the conduct is intended or very likely to bring about the death of a person. It generally is agreed that no one should have the capacity to consent to conduct intended or very likely to bring about their death, or intended to bring about physical invasion of his or her person that is likely to result in death, except when undertaken for medical reasons.

Because AIDS is likely to be fatal and because HIV is susceptible to transmission through the shared use of needles, an intravenous drug user who knows that he or she has contracted AIDS may be subject to tort liability despite the consent of the other party sharing the needles. In addition, when there is a showing of intentional transmission or gross disregard of the likelihood of transmission of HIV, a survivor may maintain a suit for wrongful death against the person inducing or assisting another to engage in drug use with contaminated needles.

5. Contributory Negligence

Contributory negligence is conduct on the part of the plaintiff, sufficiently connected to the harm suffered to constitute a legal cause thereof, that falls below the standard to which the plaintiff is required to conform for his or her own protection. A reason for denying the plaintiff recovery is that his or her own conduct is the proximate cause of the injury, *i.e.*, the plaintiff's negligence is an independent intervening cause between the defendant's negligence and the resultant harm. In determining whether a plaintiff is contributorily negligent, the plaintiff is judged by the same standard of conduct as the defendant: that of the reasonable person of ordinary prudence under like circumstances. Contributory negligence may consist not only of a failure to discover or to appreciate a risk that would be apparent to a reasonable person, or of a mistake in dealing with it, but also of an intentional but unreasonable exposure to a danger of which the plaintiff is aware.

At common law, contributory negligence was a total bar to a plaintiff's recovery. In recent years, many states have adopted a scheme of comparative negligence that changes the effect that a plaintiff's negligence has on recovery. Instead of barring all recovery, it reduces the total amount of the plaintiff's damages in proportion to his or her negligence. A person who shares the unsterilized needles of another almost certainly departs from the standard of conduct of a reasonable person, given the widespread understanding of the danger of becoming infected with HIV or of contracting AIDS from the sharing of needles and the relative ease with which persons may protect themselves.

6. Assumption of Risk

The defense of assumption of risk requires a showing that the plaintiff voluntarily incurred a known risk that resulted in his or her injury. To establish assumption of risk on the part of a plaintiff, it is necessary to show that the plaintiff knew that the risk was present, understood its nature, and freely and voluntarily incurred the risk.

A principal context in which a plaintiff is said to have assumed a risk is where he or she is aware of a risk that already has been created by the negligence of the defendant and voluntarily chooses to proceed to encounter the risk. A similar situation is the one in which the plaintiff is provided with some item that he or she knows is unsafe and proceeds to use it anyway. In most cases in which a person voluntarily accepts the use of the needles of another drug user or shares his or her own needles with another, that person can be said to have assumed the risk of being infected with HIV or of contracting AIDS as a result of shared-needle use.

One significant factor in determining assumption of risk is the actual knowledge and understanding of the plaintiff with regard to the risk of contracting AIDS as a result of shared-needle use. Unlike the standard of care for measuring a plaintiff's contributory negligence, which is the objective standard of the reasonable and prudent person, the standard of knowledge for assumption of risk is a subjective one related to the particular plaintiff and his or her situation. The age, experience, and ability to comprehend the risk in a situation will be taken into account to determine if the plaintiff consented to assume the risk of infection from shared-needle use. If a plaintiff is immature or mentally impaired, he or she may be found not to have the competence to consent to assume the risk and the person providing or sharing needles who transmits HIV through such needle use may remain liable.

Finally, the plaintiff must freely and voluntarily participate in the sharing of needles for drug use before he or she can be said to have assumed the risk of contracting AIDS from this activity. In some cases, a person may be said not to have assumed a risk where they relied on the judgment of another person or an assurance that a situation was safe. However, where the danger is so obvious that there can be no reasonable reliance upon such an assurance, a person will be found to have assumed the risk no matter what assurances may have been given. An adult with knowledge of the danger of contracting AIDS from shared-needle use may decide to rely on the initial user's assurance that he or she is free from HIV infection. In most instances, such reliance will fail to prevent successful assertion of the assumption of risk defense.

E. CHILD BIRTH

HIV can be transmitted from infected women to their fetuses during pregnancy, labor, and delivery. The risk of perinatal transmission from an infected mother is about 30%. As such, although the risk of transmission is real, it is not inevitable.

A child born with AIDS will necessarily suffer from the disease and may die from it. In addition, there are many extraordinary medical expenses associated with care and treatment. Suits may be brought in the name of the child (and in some cases in the parent's own right) against an infected parent or sexual partner of the mother and, in certain instances, against those responsible for supplying infected blood or blood products.

1.   Suit for Prenatal Injury

A child born alive may maintain an action in every jurisdiction for prenatal injuries. If the child dies as a result of such injuries after birth, an action can be maintained by his or her survivor for wrongful death. The more difficult question arises as to whether claims should be permitted where the harmful contact with the mother occurs before the child is conceived. In the malpractice context, some courts have found liability for preconception injuries resulting from negligent injury to the mother some years before conception.

A supplier of blood who has been negligent in providing a woman with HIV-contaminated blood before or during pregnancy is probably liable to a subsequently born child for injuries resulting from transmission of the virus and for the ultimate contraction of AIDS. In *Renslow v. Mennonite Hospital*, the Illinois Supreme Court considered the question of whether a child, not conceived at the time of negligent acts related to a blood transfusion, could maintain a cause of action against a physician and a hospital for the ultimate injuries resulting from the negligence.

The defendants had negligently transfused the plaintiff's mother with incompatible blood when the mother was a teenager. The mother had no immediate adverse reaction from the transfusion and did not learn that her blood had been sensitized until eight years later when she was pregnant. As a result of the mother's blood having been sensitized, the child suffered permanent damage to various organs, including its brain and central nervous system. Even though the negligent conduct occurred prior to conception, the court held that it was foreseeable that a teenage girl would later bear a child who would be injured by an improper blood transfusion. The court found that the availability of medical techniques that would have eliminated the harm caused by the defendants' negligence justified the placing of responsibility on the defendants.

Health care providers whose malpractice in the course of treating a pregnancy necessitates a blood transfusion can be held liable for associated harm if the blood was tainted with HIV. In *Gaffney v. United States*, the plaintiff, a member of the United States Marine Corps, alleged that the defendant's negligence in the management of his wife's pregnancy in 1981 caused her to require a transfusion, which resulted in her infection with HIV. As a result, a subsequently conceived child and the plaintiff contracted HIV. The plaintiff's wife and the child later died of AIDS. The plaintiff brought his action under the Federal Tort Claims Act on behalf of himself, his deceased wife, and child, and as guardian of his daughter, who was the only member of the family to escape HIV infection. A federal district court held that the defendant was negligent in the treatment of the plaintiff's wife, that she required a transfusion as a direct result of this negligence, that it was foreseeable in 1981 that a communicable disease could be transmitted through a blood transfusion, and that liability extended to all affected family members.

2. Parent-Child Immunity

At one time, courts refused to allow an action between a minor child and a parent for personal torts, regardless of whether the torts were intentional or negligent. Some courts, however, allowed recovery for personal injuries that were intentionally inflicted, and several extended liability to "willful or wanton" or reckless conduct.

Since 1963, more than half the states have abrogated parent-child immunity either by judicial decision or statute. Some courts have gone so far as to hold parents liable for negligent or intentional prenatal injury to a child; for example, liability has been recognized where a mother ingested drugs that caused her child to be born with a deformity.

There is authority to hold a parent liable who transmits HIV to a child during pregnancy, and possibly for conduct prior to conception that ultimately results in transmission of the virus to the child. Thus, a mother who engages in intravenous drug use with shared needles may be liable to a child for transmission of the virus. Likewise, a father who knows that he is infected with HIV, but engages in sexual intercourse and transmits the virus to the mother, may be held liable for the foreseeable transmission of the HIV virus to the child and for the child's ultimate development of AIDS.

3. Wrongful Birth and Wrongful Life

The theory of wrongful birth applies when the parents of a disabled child bring a claim on their own behalf for the expense of caring for their child, as well as the pain and suffering they experience as a result of being denied the opportunity to decide whether to avoid giving birth. In order to prevail on such a theory, the parents must establish that they would have avoided conception or terminated the pregnancy had they been properly advised of the risk of birth defects to the potential child.

A claim for wrongful life applies when the impaired child brings suit on his or her own behalf alleging that but for the physician's or health care provider's negligent advice to the parents or negligent treatment of the mother, he or she would not have been born with an impairment. In other words, the child claims the defendant wrongfully deprived the parents of information that would have prevented the child's birth and that the child was a foreseeable victim of such wrongful deprivation of information.

Wrongful birth and wrongful life claims generally arise when a health care provider fails to accurately inform, advise, counsel, or provide proper testing or medical care to the child's parents concerning genetic or other conditions likely to result in the impairment of a child. In those jurisdictions that have allowed a wrongful life cause of action, plaintiffs have been able to recover only special damages, *i.e.*, extraordinary expenses for medical care incurred over the child's lifetime, and have not been able to recover general damages.

Since the risk of prenatal transmission of HIV from an infected mother is high, physicians may be liable for not offering HIV antibody testing to a pregnant woman. Where a woman can show that she was known by a physician to be at risk for HIV infection, was not offered HIV antibody testing by the physician that would have revealed that she was infected, and would have aborted her fetus had she been informed of her HIV infection, a claim for wrongful birth will lie in those jurisdictions that recognize such a cause of action. Moreover, in the minority of jurisdictions that permit a wrongful life cause of action, suit can be brought in the child's own right for damages for the costs and burdens associated with HIV infection.

F. MEDICAL MALPRACTICE AND LIABILITY

A physician-patient relationship is normally a prerequisite to a medical malpractice suit against a physician. The liability of health care providers is governed by general negligence principles. Malpractice can be defined as unskilled practice resulting in injury to a patient or as a failure to exercise the required degree of care, skill, and diligence appropriate under the circumstances. The duty of care owed by a physician takes two forms. The first is a duty to render a quality of care consonant with the level of medical and practical knowledge the physician may reasonably be expected to possess and the medical judgment that may be expected to be exercised. The second is a duty based on the appropriate use of the medical facilities, services, equipment, and options that are reasonably available.

1. Diagnosis

Failure to diagnose a patient's HIV-related condition is actionable if such a failure leads to delay in treatment, to a lack of treatment, or to an incorrect treatment. In the context of HIV infection, a failure to diagnose may result in a patient failing to receive available medication directed at the virus itself. A failure to diagnose an underlying HIV infection may lead a physician to prescribe medicine that, although appropriate for the opportunistic condition in the absence of HIV infection, further depresses the immune system and results in a worsening of the HIV-infected patient's prospects.

Incorrect treatment or unnecessary treatment often results from an incorrect diagnosis. Most state courts have recognized that merely subjecting a patient to a medical or surgical treatment that is unnecessary is a sufficient basis for recovery of damages.

HIV infection is associated with certain clinical features, such as persistent generalized lymphadenopathy. In addition, certain laboratory findings may support a diagnosis, such as leukopenia and lymphopenia. Failure to identify relevant clinical symptoms or to order appropriate laboratory tests may give rise to an incorrect diagnosis for which a physician may be liable if incorrect treatment decisions are made on the basis of such errors.

2. Treatment Decisions

Incorrect or inadequate treatment may give rise to liability on the part of a physician. A physician is obligated to use that degree of skill and care in treating the patient as would be exercised by the average reputable physician. Earlier cases held a physician to the standards of care of physicians practicing in the local community. Increasingly, however, courts are holding physicians to the standard of care exercised by physicians of a given specialty throughout the country. In the AIDS context, physicians are likely to be held to a national standard of care because medical societies and health care associations are making the latest developments in treatment alternatives widely available through scientific publications and educational programs.

A physician is not required to guarantee a cure or improvement in a patient's condition. A physician does agree to use the diligence and exercise the ordinary skill of a physician in his or her specialty. However, no inference of negligence can be drawn from the fact that a patient dies or the condition of the patient does not improve.

Where established treatments are or have been less than successful and the patient's condition is sufficiently serious, a physician may consider using experimental treatments. If the physician can justify innovative techniques or therapies as being in the best interest of the patient and not simply an opportunity to obtain research information, and so long as the physician receives informed consent, the physician will not subsequently be deemed as having acted in a legally negligent manner.

3. Infection

Physicians and health care providers have a duty to protect patients from injury due to infections. Liability arises upon a showing of unsanitary conditions, such as improperly sterilized instruments, and a showing of a causal relationship between the condition and the alleged injury. For example, a patient was able to recover where the evidence showed that the plaintiff had been placed in a semi-private room with a patient who exhibited symptoms of a staphylococcus infection.

A physician has been held liable for patients' infections where the physician failed to sterilize instruments, or failed to wash his or her hands before performing a medical procedure. Similarly, a blood donation center may be liable in negligence where a donor is infected as a result of failure to maintain sterile techniques during blood donation.

Every state has regulations and standards with respect to infection control. In Illinois, for example, the applicable regulations set forth separate requirements for sterilization of equipment, instruments, utensils, water, and supplies. A violation of such regulations that results in the patient becoming infected will lead to liability. A hospital's failure to comply with a licensing regulation requiring the segregation of sterile and non-sterile needles has been held to constitute evidence of negligence.

A hospital also may be liable for failing to screen its personnel for an infectious disease. Liability has been imposed on a hospital for an inadequate screening program where it failed to give a pre-employment examination, including a nose and throat culture, to a nurse assigned to a newborn nursery. The nurse subsequently infected an infant with a staphylococcus infection. In another case, a hospital was held liable for its negligence in assigning a tubercular nurse, who had a chronic cough and cold, to attend a newborn infant. The infant later contracted tuberculosis and died.

In the AIDS context, there is a need to sterilize equipment lest it serve as a means of transmitting the virus from one patient to another. Since HIV is not transmitted through casual contact with health care personnel, concern properly focuses on those physicians and health care workers who are infected with HIV and engage in invasive procedures that may facilitate blood-to-blood contact between patient and health care personnel.

G. DEFAMATION

Defamation is an untrue written (libel) or oral (slander) communication to someone other than the subject that tends to injure the claimant's reputation. A qualified privilege exists for a good faith publication made in relation to carrying out a public or private duty. This principle is reflected in the case of *Simonsen v. Swenson*, which involved disclosures by a physician that a patient had a venereal disease. The Nebraska Supreme Court held that a qualified privilege exists when a defendant can show that the disclosure is necessary to prevent the spread of disease, that the communication is to one whom it is reasonable to suppose might otherwise be exposed, and that the defendant acted in good faith, with reasonable grounds for disclosure, and without malice.

The difficulty in obtaining recovery in an action for defamation is illustrated by the New York case of *France v. St. Clare's Hospital and Health Center*. The plaintiff alleged defamation on the basis of a letter to his brother for whom the plaintiff was making a directed blood donation. The letter falsely reported that the plaintiff's blood had tested positive for a venereal disease. A New York state appellate court acknowledged that at common law false imputation of a venereal disease was libelous *per se,* and actionable without the necessity of proving any actual damage. Nevertheless, the court found that constitutional concerns had eroded the law of defamation so that, absent proof of actual damages resulting from harm to the plaintiff's reputation, the plaintiff could not recover on a claim of defamation unless he could prove actual malice.

Despite the difficulties faced by a plaintiff who wishes to bring a defamation suit, the plaintiff in *McCune v. Neitzel* succeeded in winning a $25,000 judgment on the ground that the defendant had spread a false rumor that he had AIDS. According to the plaintiff, a twenty-seven year old single man, he became depressed, started drinking, gained weight, and was shunned by his friends and neighbors after the defendant stated that he had AIDS. In rejecting the defendant's request for a new trial, the Nebraska Supreme Court found that the defendant had slandered the plaintiff, rejected her contention that she had not meant her statement to become public knowledge, and reversed the trial judge's decision to grant the defendant a new trial on damages on the ground that the jury had been influenced by passion and prejudice in awarding the plaintiff the amount that it had.

H. INVASION OF PRIVACY

An actionable invasion of privacy occurs when there is a public disclosure of private facts that would be highly offensive to a person of reasonable sensibilities and there is no legitimate interest that favors release of the information. It is important to note that disclosure of information about another's HIV status will be deemed reasonable under certain circumstances. Even where disclosure is clearly unreasonable, however, a plaintiff is likely to be confronted with several formidable obstacles.

A question of liability for invasion of privacy might arise because of publication in a periodical or in the media that a person has AIDS or is HIV-infected. One of the primary limitations placed on the right of privacy is that it does not prohibit the publication of matters that are of legitimate public or general interest. Courts increasingly take the position that at some point the public interest in obtaining information becomes dominant over the individual's desire for privacy. Given the widespread reporting of AIDS as a cause of death in newspaper obituaries and the publication of medical facts related to the treatment of individuals such as Rock Hudson before his death, it is likely that a defendant will be able to establish a public interest in an HIV infection or AIDS diagnosis reported in a newspaper or by the media.

A second situation in which a claim for invasion of privacy is likely to be raised is where an individual informs others of the HIV status of the plaintiff in order to warn others of the danger of infection, especially from sexual relations with that party. Precedent has long existed recognizing the right of a physician to disclose to a patient's spouse that the patient has a venereal disease. A California statute specifically provides immunity from prosecution for a physician disclosing a patient's HIV status to a third party believed to be the patient's spouse. On the other hand, the Illinois AIDS Confidentiality Act appears to prohibit physicians from warning third parties, including a spouse, without the patient's consent.

A number of courts have held that the constitutional right to privacy encompasses nondisclosure of one's HIV status, and that the unauthorized release of this information by government officials gives rise to liability if the plaintiff's privacy interest outweighs the government's interest in disclosure. In *Doe v. City of New York*, the New York City Commission on Human Rights issued a press release regarding a settlement of an AIDS discrimination case against an airline. The complainant, whose name was used in the press release, sued the Commission for violating his constitutional right to privacy. A federal district court in New York dismissed the privacy claim finding that the complainant had made his HIV status a matter of public record by filing a discrimination complaint with the Commission. The Second Circuit disagreed. It held that the complainant had an interest in protecting the confidentiality of his HIV status, which was not made a matter of public record by filing a discrimination complaint or entering into a conciliation agreement. The court remanded the case to determine whether the government's interest in disseminating the information outweighed the complainant's interest in protecting the confidentiality of the information.

Several courts have entertained privacy claims involving the unauthorized disclosure of HIV-related information by police officers. In *Doe v. Borough of Barrington*, for example, a federal district court held that two police officers violated the privacy rights of an HIV-positive man's wife and daughter by disclosing his serostatus to people with whom he had not had even causal contact.

I. SPECIAL PROBLEMS

1. Statutes of Repose and Statutes of Limitations

A person develops AIDS after becoming infected with HIV, but ordinarily cannot be so diagnosed until the person's body produces sufficient antibodies to be detected or until opportunistic diseases set in whose occurrence suggests the presence of HIV. The exact latency period between the initial infection with HIV and antibody development is unknown; there is a long latency between antibody development and disease outcome in those who eventually develop AIDS.

These uncertainties pose substantial barriers under statutes of repose and statutes of limitations. A statute of repose places an upper limit on the time during which an action may be commenced, and by its very nature is usually not subject to equitable tolling. In addition, because the purpose of a statute of repose is to establish certainty with respect to limitations on a tortfeasor's potential liability, the commencement of its running is usually fixed by the fairly definite time of the breach of duty and not by the plaintiff's discovery thereof or injury from the breach, either of which may occur years after the breach of duty.

Such statutes are especially troubling for the person who contracts AIDS. A diligent patient who regularly submits himself for testing may be found to be carrying HIV, but may not be susceptible to an AIDS diagnosis. When a plaintiff then files an action so as not to be barred by the statute of repose, his or her only recourse may lie in damages for emotional distress.

Even if the state's laws do not include a statute of repose, the plaintiff must still file suit within the time permitted by the appropriate statute of limitations. A statute of limitations generally bars actions not commenced within a few years of the date on which the plaintiff's cause of action accrues. Because a plaintiff's cause of action ordinarily accrues either upon discovery of the defendant's breach or upon the manifestation of injury, statutes of limitations are often less troublesome for plaintiffs than statutes of repose in cases of torts involving latent diseases. Nonetheless, their effects may be just as significant.

In some jurisdictions, the limitation period begins running at the time of the defendant's breach. For example, one court has held that the plaintiff's cause of action for asbestosis accrued on the date of his most recent exposure to the dangerous particles. While the plaintiff had no reason to suspect the disease until years after that time, nonetheless the action was held barred. In a jurisdiction following this approach, the statute of limitations is as unforgiving to plaintiffs as is a statute of repose, and in AIDS cases very often will bar recovery.

In other jurisdictions, the plaintiff's cause of action will be held to have accrued only on the date the plaintiff discovers or reasonably should have discovered the breach. While such an interpretation may provide more protection to the AIDS plaintiff than that discussed above, it may still force a plaintiff to bring an action well before any compensable or reasonably measurable harm has occurred.

The significance of the problem is illustrated by the Wyoming case of *Duke v. Housen*, in which the plaintiff discovered, well within the limitations period, that she had been infected with gonorrhea. She did not file suit until she developed serious complications as a result of the infection, which was well after the limitations period expired. The Wyoming Supreme Court held that her cause of action accrued upon her discovery of the infection and not when the most serious, and perhaps foreseeable, consequences arose.

Precisely the same problem will arise with many AIDS plaintiffs, and in effect they will be prevented from recovering for their most substantial injuries. If the alleged harm is AIDS, the latency period may preclude recovery where the statute of limitations runs from the time of the negligent act producing infection. However, if the alleged harm is the development of HIV antibodies, rather than AIDS itself, the statute of limitations may not pose a significant problem.

Two recent cases demonstrate how divided courts are on this subject. In *Doe v. American Red Cross*, an Oregon state appellate court held that the statute of limitations did not begin to run until the plaintiff actually advanced to full-blown AIDS. A few weeks later, in *Nelson v. American National Red Cross*, a federal appellate court in Washington, D.C., held that the statute of limitations began to run on the plaintiff's claim as soon as he was diagnosed as having HIV.

2. Causation

A required element to be proved in establishing tort liability for HIV transmission is causation, *i.e.*, that the defendant's breach of duty caused the injury at issue. A plaintiff must establish both cause in fact and proximate cause. Cause in fact requires a plaintiff to provide a basis for the jury to conclude that it was more likely than not that the defendant's conduct was the cause of the plaintiff's injury. Proximate cause involves a legal determination that the defendant should be held responsible for the plaintiff's injury.

Plaintiffs may use expert medical opinion to establish that a particular practice or activity, such as anal intercourse or sharing intravenous needles, is a mode of HIV transmission. However, the problem of establishing that a particular contact was the source of HIV infection requires establishing by a preponderance of the evidence that the plaintiff was not infected before the contact at issue and that the infection did not result from a subsequent contact likely to have produced infection. An easy case would involve a plaintiff who could show that he or she tested negative for HIV before contact with the defendant, has since remained monogamous and refrained from intravenous drug use, and avoided any other contact likely to have produced the infection. In such a case, the court probably would conclude that the plaintiff's injuries were caused by a breach of duty by an infected defendant.

Most suits, however, will not provide easy proof. Given the latency period for development of the antibodies to HIV, and even more significantly the latency for developing AIDS, severe practical problems will usually arise in establishing that a particular contact transmitted the disease. A person who contracts AIDS through the use of contaminated needles likely will have been involved in numerous incidents of drug use, thereby making it difficult to isolate a particular incident as the cause of the transmission. Similarly, persons with AIDS who engage in sexual activity frequently with different partners may find it insurmountably difficult to establish the causal element of the torts on which they seek to rely.

CHAPTER VII

PUBLIC HEALTH LAW

A. INTRODUCTION

Public health statutes are enacted in accordance
with specific powers invested in the government.
Federal public health legislation has been based on
a broad interpretation of the constitutional clauses
that direct the federal government to provide for
the general welfare and to regulate commerce. Under the commerce clause, the federal government
has acted in such areas as drug control, the collection of statistics, and the inclusion of AIDS as a
dangerous disease "for purposes of exclusion of
immigrants."

The public health powers of the state are extremely broad, drawing as they do on the inherent
powers of sovereignty, and are not limited to the
exercise of explicit constitutional provisions. Police
power is inherent in the exercise of sovereignty and
extends to all public needs, such as the right to pass
laws that are reasonably necessary for the protection and preservation of the peace, safety, health,
morals, and general welfare of citizens.

Constitutional law developments over the last
quarter century have placed restraints on the use of
state authority in the public health field, including

requirements of due process and the use of the least restrictive alternative available to achieve the state's legitimate purposes. Legislation that specifically addresses AIDS is subject to scrutiny in light of these constitutional developments.

States have delegated, through constitutional provisions, part of their broad power over matters of public health to county and municipal levels of government. The scope of a county's or city's public health authority is dependent on the delegation of power by the state.

The subject matter that has been dealt with through exercise of the police power in pursuit of public health is very extensive. The courts have upheld as valid the exercise of state power in almost any matter arguably related to the public's health. These include the exercise of state power to examine, treat, and quarantine in cases of contagious disease.

The seminal judicial decision in this area is *Jacobson v. Massachusetts*. In that case, the Board of Health of Cambridge had issued regulations in conformity with a state statute. The regulations required compulsory vaccination and re-vaccination of citizens for smallpox. The petitioner refused to be vaccinated and was arrested for violating the regulation. As his defense, he argued that the regulation violated due process because vaccination was against his religious beliefs and was a deprivation of his fundamental right to care for his own health. The United States Supreme Court disagreed. It held that the health board had reasonably exercised its police power in requiring the vaccinations. In reaching its decision, the Court reasoned that:

> There is, of course, a sphere within which the individual may assert the supremacy of his own will and rightfully dispute the authority of any human government, especially of any free government existing under a written constitution, to interfere with the exercise of that will. But, it is equally true that in every well-ordered society charged with the duty of conserving the safety of its members, the rights of the individual in respect of his liberty may at times, under the pressure of great danger be subjected to such restraints, to be enforced by reasonable regulations, as the safety of the general public may demand.

Compulsory medical examinations and treatment have been upheld. For example, courts have approved statutes requiring vaccination prior to school attendance, compulsory examination of people applying for a marriage license, pre-employment testing for contagious disease in occupations where the applicant will be dealing with the public, and compliance with sanitation laws in private and public buildings.

Another broad police power of the state is the authority to involuntarily institutionalize individuals under certain circumstances. The two existing forms of exercise of this power most relevant to AIDS are involuntary hospitalization of the mentally ill and institutionalization of drug abusers.

The major limitation on the exercise of the state's public health authority are constraints found in the federal and state constitutions. Constitutional limitations involve both procedural and substantive rights that effectively limit the exercise of the state's police power. The substantive right of privacy first articulated in *Griswold v. Connecticut* places limits on the exercise of the state's police power. In *Griswold*, the United States Supreme Court invalidated state restrictions on the use of contraceptives on the ground that such regulations violate the zone of privacy between married people. This right has been extended to include the use of contraceptives by unmarried persons and by minors. In determining the constitutionality of the regulations at issue in these cases, the Court has required the state not only to show that the regulations are reasonable, but also that they are justified by a compelling state interest. The right of privacy decisions have generally involved issues of reproduction; their applicability to the full range of public health law remains uncertain.

A second limitation on the exercise of the state's police power is the required use of the least restrictive alternative available when limiting an individual's liberty in pursuit of a valid state interest. The required use of the least restrictive alternative has been extensively developed in the context of civil commitment proceedings. This requirement represents a balancing of the liberty interests of the individual with the interest of society. The "balancing of interests" requirement reflects the fact that public health regulations involving involuntary institutionalization are an exercise of the police power resulting in a form of preventive detention that necessarily involves a deprivation of personal liberty. Any public health measures restricting the liberty of HIV-infected patients must be scrutinized to ensure compliance with the least restrictive alternative standard.

Procedural limitations on the exercise of the state's public health powers derive from the due process clause of the Fifth Amendment, which prohibits the federal government from depriving any person of life, liberty, or property without due process of law, and the Fourteenth Amendment, which imposes on the states a nearly identical obligation of due process. In most state constitutions there is a similar requirement that the state provide its citizens with due process of law. Due process requires that the government use fundamentally fair procedures in exercising its police power. While rigorous procedural requirements have been imposed in criminal cases, courts scrutinize the procedures in civil cases less carefully.

Although the specific requirements of a fundamentally fair procedure depend on the type of proceeding and the issue under consideration, general principles of due process require notice to the person involved, some type of hearing, and the right to representation by counsel. The procedural due process required in administrative or judicial proceedings involving enforcement of HIV-related regulations will vary both by the type of proceeding and the liberty issue at stake. Perhaps the best analogies are to be drawn to cases in the mental health field and cases involving juvenile authorities, where courts have given the fullest consideration of procedural due process in civil proceedings.

Three principal approaches have been taken in dealing statutorily with AIDS: treating AIDS as a communicable disease, treating AIDS as a sexually transmitted disease, and treating AIDS by means of specific legislation. The public health techniques used to combat the spread of HIV infection include: education, testing and counseling, reporting and contact tracing, and quarantine, isolation, and regulation of public places. In order to obtain citizen cooperation and compliance, a rigorous scheme of confidentiality of AIDS-related records has been developed in some states.

B. DRUG DEVELOPMENT

From the beginning of the HIV epidemic, issues relating to drug development have been a source of both hope and frustration to the thousands of people affected by HIV. AIDS activists early on protested that the federal government's drug development and testing process were overly-bureaucratic and moved too slowly to develop protocols and get drugs into trials. As a result of these protests, the FDA, as part of its review of new drugs, made an adjustment in its rating system that moves all HIV-related drugs ahead of other products.

Clinical drug trials are conducted for the purpose of scientifically testing the safety and efficacy of experimental drugs before they are marketed. Traditionally, these trials have involved the fewest number of people necessary to obtain reliable data, thus minimizing the impact of any harmful side effects. However, because of the fatal nature of AIDS, access to drug trials has been expanded in order to determine more rapidly the value of particular drugs and to provide hope and the possibility of treatment to the thousands of people with HIV.

The FDA also has developed other mechanisms to increase the availability of HIV-related drugs, including treatment INDs and "community-based" trials. Treatment INDs permit physicians to prescribe an experimental drug while it is being tested in a clinical trial. This is a vital tool for moving HIV-related drugs to larger patient populations. AZT, the first approved antiviral therapy for HIV infection, initially was made available under a treatment IND. The cost of HIV-related drugs remains an issue of particular concern. When AZT was initially approved, it cost each patient $8,000–10,-000 per year, making it the most expensive drug ever marketed. AIDS patients successfully challenged the early refusal of some states to cover AZT by arguing that it was a "medically necessary" treatment.

C. AIDS EDUCATION

AIDS education has been a principal instrument for combatting the spread of HIV infection. Educational programs are targeted to four populations: the general public, school and college-age persons, persons at increased risk, and health care workers. The principal methods used in AIDS education have been: television and radio (including public service announcements and news coverage), newspapers (including feature stories, news coverage, and advertisements), posters (including billboards and bus signs), printed materials (including brochures, newsletters, and resource materials), live presentations (including workshops and outreach activities at bars, baths, bookstores, and on the streets), and counseling, testing, and referral of sex and needle-sharing partners.

The general public needs AIDS education to develop an understanding of the problems raised by the disease and to support prevention efforts. AIDS education in schools and colleges provides information about sexually transmitted diseases and drug abuse to individuals at a time when they have the greatest curiosity about such matters. Uninfected persons whose behavior or circumstances puts them at increased risk are targeted for special education programs. Finally, there is a particular need for outreach and education for health care personnel whose work puts them at risk of HIV infection.

Many states mandate AIDS education in public schools, and it has been estimated that 93% of all public high schools now offer courses that deal with AIDS. The statutory mandate to provide AIDS education in the schools has taken different forms:

as part of comprehensive health education courses on sexually transmitted disease, as part of sex education on communicable disease, and as part of the health curriculum as special AIDS education.

Parents in some districts have opposed AIDS education programs on the ground that they violate their right to the free exercise of religion. As a result of this opposition, many statutes restrict the type of prevention education that is offered to students. For example, a number of statutes require that abstinence be stressed as the best way to prevent HIV transmission. Illinois' statute requires that course materials and teaching "honor monogamous, heterosexual marriage." A number of statutes permit parents to withdraw their children from AIDS education altogether.

Some school districts have taken a more aggressive step by initiating condom distribution programs to stem the spread of HIV among students. A major controversy surrounding such programs is whether the state must secure a parent's consent before offering condoms to a minor. In *Alfonso v. Fernandez*, a New York appellate court held that New York City's condom distribution plan, which did not require parental consent or offer parents the option to "opt out," violated the substantive due process rights of parents opposed to the plan.

The court held that the condom availability component of the program was not merely educational but was a "health service" that required parental consent. Although the court found that the program violated the parents' rights to rear their children as they saw fit, it rejected the contention that the program violated the parents' free exercise of religion rights.

Public education programs directed at drug users have taken two principal forms: outreach programs to reach drug users on the streets and educational programs incorporated into drug treatment programs. A typical outreach program is that developed by the New Jersey State Department of Health. It employs former drug users who have completed a methadone maintenance program and who have received intensive AIDS training. These educational programs provide a description of AIDS and the means of transmission, the need to consider drug rehabilitation treatment, the need to cease sharing drug paraphernalia, and the need to sterilize needles and syringes that are shared.

Some states have promulgated legislative directives that require state agencies dealing with drug dependency to develop educational programs about AIDS. Typical of this legislation is the Illinois statute on alcoholism and other drug dependencies. It directs the Illinois Department of Alcoholism and Drug Abuse to develop AIDS-related education and training programs for persons engaged in the treatment and detoxification of alcoholics and drug addicts. The department also is directed to include an educational component to inform participants in treatment programs of the causes, means of transmission, and methods available to reduce the risk of acquiring or transmitting AIDS.

D. NEEDLE EXCHANGE PROGRAMS

To curb the spread of HIV among intravenous drug users, several states and cities have established needle exchange programs that offer drug users AIDS education, clean syringes, sterilizing bleach, general AIDS education, and pamphlets describing how to disinfect drug paraphernalia. Advocates of needle exchange programs claim that the scarcity of sterile syringes drives drug users to share needles, thereby spreading HIV. Critics charge that they promote drug abuse.

The creation of a needle exchange program pursuant to a state's power to protect the public health may conflict with criminal statutes that prohibit possession or distribution of hypodermic syringes. In *Spokane County Health District v. Brockett*, the Washington Supreme Court considered whether Spokane's needle exchange program, which had been created pursuant to the state board of health's duty to prevent the spread of infectious diseases, including AIDS, violated a state statute criminalizing the distribution of drug paraphernalia. The court upheld the legality of the program, citing a statute that authorized the health department to use "appropriate materials" to control the spread of HIV.

AIDS activists in cities that do not have needle exchange programs have distributed needles to drug users in open defiance of statutes that criminalize the possession of hypodermic needles. In *People v. Bordowitz*, a group of activists who distributed needles to New York City addicts were acquitted on charges of criminal possession of hypodermic needles. The judge ruled that their conduct fell within the medical necessity defense because "when coupled with AIDS education and counselling, a needle exchange program serves as a means for convincing addicts to avoid other risk-related behavior, to get medical care and ultimately to discontinue use of drugs."

A New Jersey judge, however, expressed the adverse opinion about the consequences of needle exchange programs. In *State v. Sorge*, several defendants who had openly distributed needles, bleach, and educational pamphlets to Jersey City drug addicts were charged with criminal possession of hypodermic needles. They argued for dismissal of the charges pursuant to a statute permitting dismissal if the defendant's conduct did not actually cause or threaten the harm sought to be prevented by the applicable statute or was too trivial to warrant prosecution. The judge rejected the defense and found that the defendants' conduct had facilitated illegal drug use.

E. HIV TESTING AND COUNSELING

As explained in Chapter 1, the most common procedure to test for HIV consists of two tests performed in sequence. The first test, known as

ELISA, detects the presence of antibodies against
the major individual proteins that make up HIV. If
an initial ELISA is positive, the test is repeated. If
it is again positive, the Western blot test is performed. This sequence of tests can give an accurate
assessment of whether a person's blood contains
HIV antibodies. Individuals with confirmed test
results are presumed to be currently infected and
capable of transmitting infection through blood or
sexual contact.

1. Screening Blood and Organ Donations

Serologic testing for HIV is used for screening a
given population, such as blood donors, or for diagnosis of individual patients. The first use of HIV
antibody tests was to screen units of blood and
plasma collected for transfusion or for use in the
manufacturing of blood products.

Persons accepted as donors are informed that
their blood or plasma will be tested for HIV antibodies. If individuals indicate a preference that
their blood or plasma not be tested, they are prohibited from making donations. Donors are told that
they will be placed on the collection facility's donor
deferral list. All blood is tested for HIV antibodies
by the ELISA and no blood or plasma that is found
to be positive on initial testing is transfused or
manufactured into other products capable of transmitting infectious agents. Because of the likelihood
of a false positive result on the highly sensitive
ELISA, the test is repeated and, if positive, a confirmatory test is conducted. If the repeat ELISA test

is positive, or if other tests are positive, it is the responsibility of the collection facility to ensure that the donor is notified. These screening procedures are conducted in a manner that maintains the confidentiality of the donor's identity and test results and protects against unauthorized disclosure.

In addition to testing blood or serum in the context of blood donation, the PHS has recommended that the blood or serum of donors of organs, tissue, or semen intended for human use be similarly tested and that the test result be used to evaluate the appropriate use of such material from these donors. The organs, tissue, and semen obtained from HIV-positive persons are considered potentially infectious.

2. Testing Patients

HIV testing is regarded as appropriate in connection with the diagnosis and treatment of a patient. More controversial is the desire to use HIV testing as a patient screening device to alert health care personnel of the need to follow procedures to reduce the risk of HIV transmission. The CDC and other public health authorities have opposed the general screening of patients for HIV. Instead, the CDC has recommended implementation of universal precautions for infection control that result in treating all patients as though they are HIV-positive. The OSHA has issued standards for enforcement of the CDC recommendations.

The use of HIV testing to screen patients for purposes of infection control is not forbidden by any statute. In most states, however, such testing for screening purposes can be implemented only with the patient's informed consent. Moreover, as explained in Chapter 2, the refusal to treat or care for a patient with a positive test result is likely to create liability under both federal and state anti-discrimination laws.

3. Informed Consent

Informed consent and patient autonomy provide a fundamental basis for the patient-physician relationship. This right is rooted in the constitutional right to privacy as well as common law rights to bodily integrity and individual autonomy. This basic tenet of medical ethics gives competent patients control over decisions regarding their treatment, including administration of any extraordinary diagnostic tests that may be medically indicated.

Several states have adopted statutes or regulations requiring informed consent for HIV testing in the medical context. Illinois generally requires written informed consent to HIV testing. An important exception permits physicians to test on the basis of a general consent to medical treatment. Texas permits testing without consent whenever a medical procedure is to be performed on the patient that could expose health care personnel to HIV infection.

Ordinarily, routine blood testing does not require specific consent because such tests are regarded as low risk procedures. While HIV testing does not pose any significant risk of physical injury to the vast majority of patients, the social and personal consequences of a positive HIV test militate in favor of requiring informed consent. The CDC has recommended that persons be informed before being tested for the presence of HIV.

Informed consent to HIV testing means an agreement, without inducement, to undergo the suggested tests for the presence of HIV following receipt of a fair explanation of the test. In discussing the test, the physician is expected to advise the patient of the test's purpose, potential use, and limitations. The physician also is expected to discuss the meaning of the test results, including the possibility of false positive and false negative results, as well as the procedures used in administering the test. Most experts consider physicians remiss if they fail to explain that the test is voluntary, that the patient may withdraw consent at any time, and the extent to which the law provides a right to anonymity with respect to participation in a test, disclosure of test results, and the handling of information identifying the patient and the results of the test.

Since an HIV test may have serious personal consequences for a patient, a health care provider administering such a test is well advised to obtain consent in writing on a detailed consent form.

4. Counseling

Several state statutes require counseling by a physician who orders an HIV test for a patient. For example, the law in Illinois requires pre-test counseling, including information about the meaning of the test results, the availability of additional or confirmatory testing, if appropriate, and the availability of referrals for further information or counseling.

In Florida, HIV testing requirements include pre- and post-test counseling on the meaning of a test for HIV (including the possibility of false positive or false negative results, the potential need for confirmatory testing, the social, medical, and economic consequences of a positive test result, and the need to eliminate high risk behavior). The statute also provides explicit directions for post-test counseling, which is to include face-to-face post-test counseling on the meaning of the test results, the possible need for additional testing, the social, medical, and economic consequences of a positive test result, and the need to eliminate behavior that might spread the disease to others.

It is generally agreed, whether required by statute or not, that HIV testing should be accompanied by pre- and post-test counseling. Pre-test counseling insures compliance with requirements of informed consent. Post-test counseling is needed to protect third parties, reduce the spread of HIV to others, and provide subjects with an opportunity to protect their own health.

Ethical standards require physicians and other health care providers to provide counseling to reduce the likelihood of the spread of HIV infection. Moreover, such counseling may be a significant protection from liability to third parties who are subsequently infected by a patient.

Pre-test counseling should include instruction on the nature of HIV and the means of transmission, as well as discussion of the subject's personal activities that may put themselves or others at risk. The pre-test counseling should include a discussion of the medical, psychological, and sociological implications of the HIV antibody test. Facts about the nature of the test should be discussed as part of the informed consent process.

If the test results are positive, the counselor should impart an understanding of the test, the need for discontinuing behavior likely to transmit HIV, the need for follow-up testing and care, and the availability of psychiatric services. When the result is negative, the patient must be instructed on the need to modify behavior so as to prevent future infection.

HIV testing should be made available to all who request such testing. The guidelines of the PHS give priority for testing and counseling to persons who are most likely to be infected.

5. Warning Third Parties

Court decisions from various jurisdictions have announced exceptions to the physician's duty of confidentiality. Most cases have determined that a therapist's duty to control a dangerous patient or decrease the risk of harm to the patient or a third person outweighs the confidential nature of the relationship. The landmark case authorizing a breach of confidentiality is the California Supreme Court's decision in *Tarasoff v. University of California*. In that case, the court held that a physician or a psychiatrist treating a mentally ill patient bears a duty to use reasonable care to give threatened partners such warnings as are essential to avert foreseeable danger arising from a patient's condition or treatment.

It has been argued that a physician has a duty to inform the spouse or current sexual or needle-sharing partners of an HIV-infected patient. On the other hand, if the patient has been counseled by the physician and has satisfied the physician that he or she will not engage in behavior likely to transmit HIV, the physician may not owe any further duty to third parties. Since HIV is not transmitted causally in the workplace or at home, there is no obligation to warn a patient's employer or family members other than those with whom the patient may be engaged in an activity likely to transmit the virus. Informing persons other than those at risk because of continuing sexual or needle-sharing activity with a patient would constitute a breach of confidentiality.

6. Premarital Testing

At one time, Illinois required as a pre-condition to issuance of a marriage license that the applicants obtain a medical examination, including tests to determine whether either of the parties to the proposed marriage had been exposed to HIV or any other identified causative agent of AIDS. The Illinois statute made it unlawful for a county clerk to issue a marriage license to any person who failed to present a certificate signed by the physician who administered the requisite tests. The certificate had to indicate that the tests had been administered and the results provided to the parties. It did not, however, have to indicate the test results. The Illinois law was repealed after the Illinois State Department of Public Health reported that only a very small number of positive test results had been obtained and that many state residents were avoiding testing by being married in a neighboring state.

Louisiana enacted a similar pre-marital testing law that, like the law in Illinois, subsequently was repealed. Under a Texas statute that has yet to be implemented, premarital screening for HIV infection will be required only if the seroprevalence rate among the general population increases from 0.1%, the rate at the time of enactment, to 0.83%.

Utah is the only state that has ever adopted legislation barring marriage by HIV-infected persons. A federal district court later struck down the statute on the ground that it violated the Americans with Disabilities Act. *T.E.P. v. Leavitt.*

Several states have adopted statutes that provide that applicants for a marriage license must be informed of the availability and advisability of obtaining HIV tests before marriage. Such laws do not require testing as a pre-condition to obtaining a marriage license.

A number of reasons have been given for why statutorily mandated pre-marital testing is not advisable. These include the high rate of pre-marital sex between parties seeking a marriage license, the high cost of testing, the low yield rate of persons identified as HIV-positive, the conclusion that other pre-marital screening programs have not been effective, the difficulty of keeping the test results confidential, and the relative ineffectiveness of such programs in stopping the spread of AIDS.

7. Testing Prisoners

The Federal Bureau of Prisons randomly tests all new inmates "from time to time" for HIV infection. New inmates who test negative are retested at six month intervals. Additionally, random, mandatory HIV testing of all inmates occurs on a yearly basis.

Any federal prison inmate can be ordered to undergo HIV testing if he or she: 1) has chronic symptoms suggestive of HIV infection, 2) is pregnant, 3) is receiving live vaccines, 4) is admitted to a community hospital that requires the test, or, 5) engages in "promiscuous, assaultive, or predatory sexual behavior." In addition, all inmates being considered for mandatory release, parole, or furlough in a community-based program must undergo HIV testing, although a positive test result cannot be the sole ground for an adverse decision regarding these matters. Inmates who undergo HIV testing must receive both pre- and post-test counseling. Federal prison inmates who test positive may be segregated from the general population if there is reliable evidence that they "may engage in conduct posing a health risk to another person."

The constitutionality of mandatory HIV testing and segregation of infected federal inmates has been upheld. In *Harris v. Thigpen*, for example, the Eleventh Circuit ruled that Florida's practice of screening all new inmates for HIV infection and segregating those who tested positive did not violate their constitutional right of privacy. However, while they may be tested and segregated, several courts have recognized that HIV-positive federal inmates have a constitutional right to have their HIV status kept confidential.

States have taken several approaches to testing inmates for HIV. A minority of states require mandatory HIV testing of all inmates. Other states have enacted statutes that give prison officials broad discretion to order HIV testing. Finally, a number of states require mandatory testing of every person arrested for, charged with, or convicted of certain crimes, such as sex offenses, prostitution, or intravenous drug use. Constitutional challenges to state statutes that provide for mandatory HIV testing of persons arrested for or convicted of certain crimes generally have not succeeded.

F. CONFIDENTIALITY

The level of protection of confidentiality of HIV-related medical records varies from state to state. California is representative of those states that have provided broad protection for such records. The

California statute provides that no person shall be compelled in any state or local proceeding to identify or provide characteristics that would identify any individual who is the subject of a blood test for AIDS. The statute provides for civil and criminal liability for wrongful disclosure. Other provisions provide for the confidentiality of AIDS research records by providing that research records in personal identifying form developed in the course of conducting AIDS research are confidential and not subject to discovery.

In the absence of, or in addition to specific legislation directed at protecting the confidentiality of HIV-related medical records, protection may be provided by general medical records statutes. These statutes provide an evidentiary privilege to be asserted on behalf of the patient for physician-patient communications in judicial or quasi-judicial proceedings.

Where no statutory cause of action is available, an individual whose HIV-related records have been revealed may have a cause of action for invasion of privacy. In addition, where a treating physician has breached confidentiality by unauthorized communication of HIV-related information, an action for breach of the physician-patient confidential relationship and malpractice may be available.

There are significant exceptions to the rule of confidentiality. These include communications made in the absence of a physician-patient relationship and those made for purposes other than diagnosis or treatment. A primary area where this may occur is in an employer-mandated pre-employment physical examination. Some courts have found the absence of a patient-physician relationship in such examinations. Another exception includes medical information in which there is a supervening public interest. The public is likely to be thought to have a strong interest in any data that includes information about contagious diseases.

Medical information often is collected in conformity with statutory or regulatory requirements, and may be communicated in connection with quality assurance activities to meet accreditation, regulatory, and licensing standards, or to further approved education and research programs. The patient-physician privilege may be waived either expressly or impliedly by a patient. Waiver of the privilege, for example, occurs when a patient's condition is affirmatively put into controversy in personal injury litigation. Third party payors, particularly those operating under governmental programs, have access to hospital records. Charges made for services and treatment of an HIV patient may provide a basis for inferences about a patient's diagnosis. Use of these records is restricted to purposes associated with the evaluation and audit of the health care programs.

1. Medical Records

The professional licensing laws of some states require that physicians and health care providers maintain the confidentiality of information they obtain in the course of treating their patients. Consequently, physicians and other health care providers may be found to be engaging in professional misconduct if they improperly release confidential information.

Hospitals and other facilities making unauthorized disclosures may be civilly liable where the applicable licensing statute or regulation prohibits disclosure of confidential information concerning patients. Accrediting bodies impose similar duties that require facilities to keep medical information confidential. Improper disclosure of a patient's medical records may jeopardize a facility's accreditation.

The protection given by statutes and judicial decisions are subject to a number of exceptions. One such exception is that where the supervening interest of society compels disclosure of a patient's medical information, disclosure must be made. This includes information required for birth and death certificates as well as information pertaining to infectious, contagious, or communicable disease.

2. Public Health Records

Where there is no specific AIDS confidentiality legislation in a state, AIDS-related records will be protected by general public health record confidentiality laws. If AIDS is classified as a sexually transmitted or venereal disease, records relating to AIDS have broad confidentiality protections that often include a shield from judicial subpoena. For example, until the passage of a specific AIDS confidentiality law, a New York state statute guaranteed the confidentiality of sexually transmitted disease reports, including those related to AIDS, in the possession of public health officials.

In some states, AIDS and HIV-related conditions are classified as "communicable diseases." Records of communicable diseases often do not receive the same extensive confidentiality protections as "sexually transmitted diseases." In particular, communicable disease records often are not shielded from subpoena.

3. AIDS Confidentiality Legislation and Regulations

A number of states have passed laws specifically protecting the confidentiality of HIV test results and AIDS diagnoses. Massachusetts exemplifies states with narrow disclosure limits. It prohibits HIV antibody tests without informed consent and also prohibits disclosure of test results or identification of a test subject without the written consent of the test subject.

Wisconsin law exemplifies a state with broader disclosure limits. Under Wisconsin law, test results can be disclosed without written consent from the test subject to the subject's designated health care provider, to persons procuring or distributing donated organs, to appropriate state health and other agencies, and to blood banks. The Wisconsin statute also permits providers to disclose HIV test results to health facility staff committees, groups involved in accreditation and service review, and agents or employees of the test subject's health care provider. The Wisconsin statute authorizes civil and criminal penalties for unauthorized intentional disclosure and civil liability for unauthorized negligent disclosure.

Both California and Wisconsin have statutory provisions regulating disclosure of HIV test results for research purposes. Wisconsin permits health care providers to disclose HIV test results for research purposes only if the researcher is affiliated with the patient's health care provider and has obtained clearance from an institutional review board. The researcher must also provide assurance, in writing, that the patient's identity will not be revealed, that the information will be used only for the stated research purpose, and that the identified data will not be released to persons other than those involved in the study.

None of the AIDS confidentiality statutes or regulations prohibit reporting data in compliance with public health requirements or CDC protocols. Under federal law, certain federal institutions, including the CDC, are required to assure the suppliers of research information that material that is supplied will not be used for any purpose other than that for which it was supplied unless the institution or individual supplying the information has consented to the further release of the supplied information. Confidentiality is required for all information gathered in programs receiving federal grants for AIDS prevention and surveillance.

4. Accidental Potential Exposures

Some states permit disclosure of an individual's HIV test results to members of specified groups where there has been an accidental exposure to body fluids or tissue that may permit transmission of HIV. A number of states require notification of ambulance personnel and emergency medical technicians that they have transported or treated an HIV-infected person.

Illinois permits access to a patient's HIV test results by employees of a health care provider or facility, firefighters, and emergency medical technicians who accidentally come into contact with the blood or body fluids of an individual in a manner that a physician determines might transmit HIV. The law also permits testing of a patient without informed consent when there is suspicion that a contact with the patient's blood or tissue has occurred that may have permitted HIV transmission. The statute provides that written informed consent is not required to perform a test when a health care provider, employee of a health facility, or emergency medical technician is involved in an accidental direct skin or mucous membrane contact with the blood or body fluids of an individual that is of a nature that may transmit HIV as determined by the medical judgment of a physician.

5. Confidential Health Records and Court Orders

Health care providers may be required to release medical record information pursuant to subpoena or court order. However, the question of what medical records in various contexts are open to discovery has been a matter of a great deal of litigation. For example, the Iowa Supreme Court has ruled that the identity of a potential bone marrow donor listed in a hospital's transplant registry is part of a confidential patient's record and cannot be released to a leukemia patient seeking a donor for a bone marrow transplant necessary to save his life. Most courts have refused to compel hospitals and blood banks to produce records of blood donors in AIDS-related litigation.

Courts have granted extensive protection to public health records and surveillance data. A New York appellate court refused to order the disclosure of files of the state health commissioner to litigants in a personal injury suit. The court held that the defendants were barred by the state confidentiality statute from discovery of questionnaires prepared by the public health department. The court noted, however, that the information sought could be obtained by subpoena from private sources. In doing so, the court left open the question of whether publicly collected information can be subject to compulsory disclosure if adequate circumstances favor discovery.

The very operation of AIDS-related programs may preclude discovery of records concerning participants. For example, a New York court refused to order the director of a methadone program to produce photographs of program participants on the grounds that success of such a program depends on confidentiality and participant cooperation. An Illinois appellate court denied the state's request for communicable disease reports in a criminal proceeding on the basis of state confidentiality statutes and the strong public policy favoring confidentiality in the treatment of sexually transmitted diseases.

In a case related to records of the CDC, a federal appellate court upheld the right of the CDC, which was not a party to the action, to refuse to turn over to the defendant manufacturer records identifying individuals who had participated in a CDC study of toxic shock syndrome. The defendant claimed the records were necessary to its defense in several products liability cases arising out of toxic shock injuries. The court agreed with the CDC that discovery was inappropriate because of the need for confidentiality of CDC records in order to carry out essential surveillance and epidemiological activities. However, the court indicated that there might be circumstances in which disclosure of CDC records might be ordered. Undoubtedly, the court's refusal to order the CDC to open its files was due in large part to the fact that the defendant already possessed all of the requested information except for the actual names of the participants. In fact, the CDC had revealed the names of several participants who had agreed to the release of their names to provide the defendant with information for a sample study.

The Federal Rules of Civil Procedure and virtually all state rules of civil procedure provide for the issuance of protective orders to spare a person or party from annoyance, embarrassment, oppression, or undue burden or exposure. Where discovery of AIDS-related information is ordered, a party seeking to protect the information's confidentiality may still seek protective orders governing the conditions and extent of disclosure. Protective orders may provide for *in camera* inspection of documents, impose conditions prohibiting the release of disclosed information to third parties, and impose contempt fines for breaches of confidentiality.

Some states, such as Georgia, have adopted AIDS confidentiality laws that provide that a person's seropositive status is privileged, confidential, and protected from discovery proceedings, subpoenas, and court orders. By contrast, the Illinois confidentiality statute permits disclosure of test results when there is a compelling need to know and a court order is granted after weighing such disclosure against the patient's right to privacy.

6. Discovery of Blood Donor Records

One area of litigation arising in relation to the testing of donors of blood, organs, or tissue is confidentiality and access to records of seropositivity. This issue commonly occurs when someone sues a hospital or blood bank for providing them with HIV-infected blood as a result of negligence in screening blood. The plaintiff in such cases often seeks to learn the name of the donor through discovery.

Some states have adopted confidentiality statutes protecting the identity of HIV test subjects. California has the most comprehensive confidentiality statute. It provides that no person shall be compelled in any state or local proceeding to identify or provide identifying characteristics that would identify any individual who is the subject of a blood test to detect antibodies to HIV.

The Illinois law provides very specific guidelines for court-ordered access to HIV antibody test records. A court may permit access to test results only by proof of a compelling need, not otherwise accommodated by alternative information, that outweighs the privacy interest of the test subject and the public interest in not deterring blood and organ donation. Pleadings are to substitute a pseudonym for the true name of the subject, court proceedings are to be conducted *in camera*, and if an order is issued, the court must impose appropriate safeguards against unauthorized disclosure.

It has been held in some court decisions that the identities of blood donors fall within the scope of the physician-patient privilege and are therefore not discoverable. Alternatively, it has been found that an order compelling disclosure of donor names and addresses is an unconstitutional infringement of the donor's right to privacy. Several courts have held that the disclosure of the identity of blood donors would violate state abuse-of-discovery rules. Such courts have taken the view that the public interest in an adequate volunteer blood supply outweighs any claimed benefit to the party seeking discovery.

On the other hand, some courts have permitted the discovery of the identities of blood donors. This has occurred, however, only in circumstances in which the court has been convinced that release of the information is vital and no less intrusive substitute exists. *Arnold v. American National Red Cross.*

G. REPORTING AND CONTACT TRACING

Statutes or regulations in every state require the reporting of AIDS cases to the CDC. A number of states have statutory or regulatory provisions requiring the reporting of positive HIV antibody test results with the names of the subjects. Other states require reporting of positive HIV antibody test results without personal identification of the test subject.

Information obtained from reporting of AIDS diagnoses and HIV infection have been used as the basis for epidemiologic studies and surveillance. Some states have used this information in contact tracing or partner notification programs.

1. Reporting

AIDS-related reporting requirements take three principal forms: statutes or regulations in every state that require reporting of CDC-defined cases of AIDS; specific statutory or regulatory requirements to report positive HIV antibody test results; and general statutory or regulatory provisions that do not specify HIV as reportable, but that require the reporting of any case, condition, or carrier status relating to specified communicable and sexually transmissible diseases, including AIDS.

AIDS reporting statutes and regulations have as their purposes the gathering of epidemiologic data regarding the incidence of AIDS and permitting public health action, such as contact tracing, appropriate to a specific case.

Regulatory or criminal sanctions may be sought against licensed providers who fail to comply with reporting statutes or regulations. Furthermore, a civil cause of action may be brought against a provider whose failure to report a condition required by statute or regulation to be reported results in injury to a third party by preventing implementation of a program of contact tracing or partner notification that would have enabled the third party to take action to prevent infection or to obtain effective medical treatment.

States vary in the manner in which they require the reporting of "communicable" and "sexually transmissible" diseases. California, for example, specifies by statute which diseases must be reported. On the other hand, Illinois distinguishes between communicable and sexually transmissible diseases. As to the former, Illinois simply provides the state public health department with broad powers to adopt, promulgate, repeal, and amend rules and regulations and make such investigations and inspections as it may from time to time deem necessary. This permits the state department to develop a list of reportable diseases. At one time, AIDS was designated a reportable communicable disease. Illinois now has special AIDS reporting legislation.

Whether HIV infection is categorized as a communicable or sexually transmissible disease may determine the range of measures available to public health officials to control its spread. In *New York State Society of Surgeons v. Axelrod*, four medical societies challenged the decision of the New York State Commissioner of Health to not classify HIV infection as a communicable and sexually transmissible disease. Such a classification would have triggered statutes providing for isolation, quarantine, reporting, testing, and contact tracing. The New York State Court of Appeals upheld the Commissioner's decision, finding that it was not arbitrary, capricious, or in excess of statutory authority.

Statutes or regulations in every state require reporting of CDC-defined cases of AIDS to the state health department. Several state statutes establish a registry of persons diagnosed with AIDS. A typical AIDS reporting regulation requires the following information: the individual's name, address, telephone number, age, race, ethnic background, sex, and hospital where the diagnoses was made; risk factors; diagnosis and any laboratory findings, including HIV test results; each AIDS-related opportunistic disease, such as KS, PCP, or esophageal candidiasis; and the name and address of the reporting physician.

Some states require reporting positive HIV test results. A few states, such as Colorado, require reporting of HIV test results with personal data on the test subject, including the name and address of the subject. Other states, such as Illinois, do not require the name or other identifying data concerning the test subject, but instead limit reporting to the individual's city of residence, age, race, ethic background, sex, laboratory findings, risk factors, whether the individual had previously tested positive, and whether counseling and sex partner referral have taken place.

The differences in the approaches taken by states on whether identifying information is reported represents basic policy decisions. Those states that do not require reporting of the test subject's name believe that their primary concern is epidemiological and do not wish to discourage participation in the state's voluntary testing program. States that require the reporting of the names of test subjects have justified the requirement on the grounds of needing information that will facilitate contact tracing and notifying individuals if AIDS drugs become available.

Colorado has served as a model state for evaluating the value of mandatory HIV test reporting by subject's name. It established testing centers at which individuals at risk of HIV infection are encouraged to obtain voluntary testing. Test results are maintained in a computer to enable notification for follow-up testing. The scheme has been justified by the need to have a record of infected individuals, to facilitate counseling, to monitor the spread of infection, to permit notification of positive individuals of available drug therapies, and to permit notification of negative individuals of the availability of vaccination, should it become available. There is no indication that this program has deterred voluntary testing in Colorado.

2. Contact Tracing

Contact tracing, or partner notification, has been a part of programs to control the transmission of communicable and sexually transmitted diseases for a very long time. For instance, the strategy of notifying all of the sexual partners of persons diagnosed with syphilis has been regarded as a major control measure since the 1940s. The rationale for traditional contact tracing was to treat infected individuals as early as possible in order to avoid unnecessary complications, to reduce the period of infection, and to break the transmission cycle. As treatment becomes available that interferes with HIV replication, the full range of traditional objectives may be met by contact tracing.

Opposition to contact tracing in the AIDS context has been based on several grounds: contact tracing with large, infected groups does not produce sufficient public health benefits to justify the deep invasion of privacy, contact tracing is not feasible among high-risk groups in areas of high infection, and a systematic program of contact tracing in high infection areas drains resources and is very difficult to plan and enforce.

Some contact tracing schemes provide that treating physicians directly notify the partners of their infected patients. Most programs, however, permit notification by local public health agencies. Such programs typically provide for public health department employees to approach the sexual contacts of a reported infected individual. The public health worker informs the contact that he or she may have been exposed to a specified sexually transmitted disease, such as HIV, and offers the contact the availability of testing and counseling.

The CDC has recommended notification of sexual partners of HIV-exposed individuals. Several states have adopted statutes that grant authority to public health departments to conduct contact tracing activities with information obtained voluntarily from HIV-infected individuals. Although all current contact tracing is on a voluntary basis, several state legislatures have considered bills that would have compelled disclosure of past sexual contacts.

States have taken several approaches to tracing contacts who are voluntarily identified by those who test HIV positive. Some states, such as Oregon and Maryland, have a program of notification of selected persons. These states rely on voluntary notification but provide for health department notification to persons at significant risk whom the test subject explicitly refuses to inform. Colorado is the only state employing active contact tracing that is not limited to a population group or a geographic area. Active contact tracing involves positive efforts to obtain the names of persons who have engaged in behavior likely to have facilitated HIV transmission and involves notification of all contacts identified by any HIV-infected person.

A number of states have enacted laws mandating notification of persons who have been in contact with HIV-infected persons where there may have been exposure to infected blood or tissue. Most of these statutes require the health care facility or treating physician to notify specified personnel if a patient is determined to be HIV-positive. Personnel to be notified usually include emergency medical technicians, paramedics, and ambulance personnel. Firefighters and police often are listed as well.

A major concern related to contact tracing is the confidentiality of public health records. To date, public health officials appear to have done a good job in preserving the confidentiality of information received in the implementation of contact tracing programs.

3. Death Reporting

Some states have statutes requiring notification to medical examiners, funeral directors, embalmers, and others handling or disposing of human bodies that the individual died with an AIDS diagnosis or was HIV-infected. Such notice is intended to facilitate compliance with proper infection control procedures when handling the body of an HIV-infected person. The health care provider releasing the body is often given the responsibility of notifying the proper parties. Some states require written notification of an AIDS diagnosis or HIV infection.

Others require notification where the disease is known or suspected. The CDC does not recommend tagging bodies of HIV-infected persons to enable special precautions with such a body, but instead recommends that morticians and others handling bodies follow universal precautions to protect against infection.

Every state requires the reporting of deaths with a medical certificate describing the cause of death. Death certificates usually report both the immediate cause of death, such as PCP, as well as the ultimate cause of death, such as AIDS. Some state statutes make death certificates public records, while some courts have found confidentiality protections do not extend to death certificates. In *Tri-State Publishing Co. v. City of Port Jervis*, a New York state trial court held that a copy of a death certificate of a hospital patient believed to have died from AIDS had to be turned over by the city to a newspaper. The court concluded that the document was not privileged under state law nor exempt from access for privacy considerations.

H. CONTROL MEASURES

1. Quarantine

Quarantine law based on "status," as discussed here, is to be distinguished from quarantine based on "behavior," which in this book is termed "isolation." The power to quarantine persons with communicable diseases is provided for by statute in every state and by federal statute. Some states

have enacted statutes that specifically extend quarantine or isolation authority to persons with AIDS
or HIV infection. State and federal courts have
upheld the enforcement of quarantine statutes as a
valid exercise of the state's police power. In *Jacobson v. Massachusetts*, the United States Supreme
Court upheld a conviction for refusal to submit to
smallpox vaccination. The Court broadly held that
states have the authority to enact quarantine laws
and health laws as a means of protecting a community against communicable disease.

State and federal courts regularly have upheld
state quarantine statutes directed at communicable
diseases. For example, in *People ex rel. Barmore v.
Robertson*, the Illinois Supreme Court upheld an
Illinois law providing for quarantine of individuals
believed to be a threat to the general public. The
plaintiff, a person infected with typhoid, filed a writ
of habeas corpus claiming that she had been unlaw-
fully restrained. The court upheld the act of re-
straining the plaintiff, who ran a boarding house
where several boarders had become infected with
typhoid, and also approved the decision to quarantine the house, on the grounds that both were
proper exercises of the state's police power.

Quarantine of persons with venereal disease also
has been upheld. For the most part, quarantine of
persons with venereal disease has been aimed at
prostitutes. In *Reynolds v. McNichols*, a prostitute
brought a civil rights action challenging a hold-and-
treat ordinance. The Tenth Circuit upheld the
ordinance as a valid use of the state's police power.

The ordinance in question provided that one suspected of being infected with a venereal disease could either be detained for examination for forty-eight hours or could take medication and be immediately released.

HIV-infected female prostitutes have been quarantined in California, Florida, and Nevada. In one Florida case, a female prostitute with AIDS was confined to her home and ordered to wear an electronic transmitter that signaled police if she traveled more than two hundred feet from her telephone.

Quarantine of AIDS-infected prisoners has been upheld in New York. In *LaRocca v. Dalsheim*, a state trial court upheld a Department of Correctional Facilities regulation under which HIV-infected prisoners were segregated from other prisoners in order to halt the transmission of HIV. The court held that the corrections authorities had acted reasonably in their attempt to stop HIV transmission. Although the court found that quarantine was appropriate in the prison context, it expressed the view that medical knowledge about HIV suggested that mass quarantine of the general public infected with HIV would not be justified.

Courts continue to hold that isolating HIV-infected inmates does not violate the Eighth or Fourteenth amendments. *Harris v. Thigpen*. Additionally, one court has held that the federal government did not violate an inmate's Eighth Amendment rights by housing him with an inmate who was dying of AIDS. *Johnson v. United States*. The segregation of HIV-infected inmates, however, may violate AIDS confidentiality laws or the right to privacy if isolation in itself automatically reveals their HIV status to others.

There are many reasons why general isolation of HIV-infected persons is not reasonable: the sheer number of people capable of transmitting the virus (which is estimated to be close to two million), the fact that there is no finite period of infectiousness so that any isolation is potentially without limit as to time, the fact there is no prevention or curative treatment so that those isolated must remain so permanently, and the fact that the virus is not spread through casual contact. Each of these facts makes quarantine based on status unnecessary and excessively restrictive.

2. Isolation

Isolation, or quarantine based on behavior, imposes restrictions on those HIV-infected persons whose actions are likely to facilitate transmission of HIV. Several states have enacted statutes that are directed at recalcitrant individuals with HIV infection who persist in behaviors likely to transmit HIV.

For example, regulations of the Illinois Department of Public Health provide for isolation of noncompliant HIV carriers. Such carriers are defined as persons who know or have reason to know that they are infected with HIV and are engaging in conduct or activities that place others at risk of exposure to HIV infection as a result of specified behaviors. The specified behaviors include: selling or donating blood, sperm, organs, or other tissues or bodily fluids; engaging in or attempting, offering, or soliciting sexual activities likely to transmit HIV; sharing intravenous drug needles with another person; or actions or statements by an individual that are clear indicators of his or her intention to place others at risk of exposure to HIV infection, such as a statement of intent to perform a specific action in order to infect another person.

Such statutes generally include two important features: a showing that isolation is the least restrictive alternative available (i.e., that the alternative of isolation is one of last resort), and a requirement of a court order making the findings necessary to permit the respective department of public health to impose isolation.

For example, a Colorado statute authorizes the imposition of specified restrictive measures or orders on individuals with HIV infection only when all other efforts to protect the public health have failed. The statute further provides that orders and measures are to be applied serially, with the least intrusive measure utilized first. The burden of proof is on the state or local health department to show that specific grounds exist for the issuance of orders or measures and that the terms are no more restrictive than necessary to protect the public health. Similarly, an Oregon statute requires isolation to be the least restrictive alternative necessary to protect the public health and requires compliance with detailed due process provisions and issuance of a court order.

A significant feature of the Illinois regulations governing isolation of non-compliant HIV carriers is the limiting of the order of isolation to the period for which the individual refuses to cease engaging in the behavior likely to transmit HIV. The regulations provide for obtaining a court order isolating such person in a restricted environment until such time as he or she has demonstrated a willingness and ability, as shown by reported acts and statements of intention, to refrain from behavior that places others at risk of exposure to HIV infection.

The Presidential Commission on the Human Immunodeficiency Virus Epidemic recommended that states adopt statutes authorizing the isolation of non-compliant HIV-infected persons. However, the Commission recommended that less restrictive measures should be exhausted before more restrictive measures, such as limited isolation, are imposed. Further, the Commission recommended that in exercising powers of isolation, there should be a heavy burden of proof requiring a showing that such measures are necessary and appropriate and that a factual basis exists for making the determination to isolate an individual.

3. Regulation of Places

Certain public places, such as bathhouses and bookstores with video booths, are locales in which high-risk sexual activity may occur. Some states have enacted statutes that specifically prohibit the operation of bathhouses. In other states, public health officials have sought to close such establishments under regulations adopted pursuant to their statutory authority to act to protect the public health. For example, the New York State Public Health Council passed a regulation defining anal intercourse and fellatio as high risk sexual activity and provided that no establishment would be permitted to accommodate persons engaging in such activity on the premises. The regulation was the basis for closing a gay bar and a gay bathhouse. The order against the gay bathhouse was upheld on constitutional and statutory grounds. *City of New York v. New St. Mark's Baths.*

Using a least restrictive approach, a state trial court in San Francisco refused to grant the city's petition for an injunction to close all of the bathhouses in the city. Instead, the court ordered the proprietors of the bathhouses to prohibit high-risk sexual activity, enjoined the bathhouse from renting private rooms, required the doors to individual cubicles, booths, and rooms to be removed, and mandated a program of safe sex education.

The approach of eliminating structures that promote anonymous sexual activity rather than closing establishments where such activity has occurred was approved by the Seventh Circuit in *Berg v. Health and Hospital Corp. of Marion County.* The case involved a city ordinance that sought to prevent the spread of HIV by requiring "open booths" for individuals viewing films. The appeals court found that the ordinance, as applied to a bookstore with video booths, was constitutional. It held that the measure was narrowly tailored because, as other courts had observed, the open booth regulation appeared to be the least burdensome means of controlling illegal activity within the booths. The court declined to speculate as to other possible alternatives the agency might have employed, noting that the plaintiff had not identified any less restrictive alternatives and expressing doubts that any such alternatives existed. Finally, the court found that the ordinance was neither overbroad nor vague, since it was plainly directed at those establishments that provided individual booths where high-risk sexual activity could occur. The court concluded that the ordinance was a valid and constitutional regulation serving a legitimate governmental interest.

Constitutional attacks on regulatory measures directed at gay bathhouses where anal intercourse or fellatio occur are not likely to be successful. The United States Supreme Court in *Bowers v. Hardwick* held that private homosexual activity between consenting adults in their own home is not constitutionally protected. If the state can punish such activity when it occurs in a private home, it clearly can regulate such activity in public places as well as in those facilities where such activity occurs.

I. MENTAL HEALTH CARE

AIDS patients often manifest psychological disturbances associated with the physiological impact of infection, including depression, confusion, anger, and despair. It is important to distinguish AIDS mood disturbances, which are to be expected, from clinical psychiatric syndromes that may require therapeutic interventions. A major depression or anxiety disorder that may be amenable to treatment with conventional psychopharmacological agents should not be mistaken for the fear and despondency that occur in connection with an AIDS diagnosis.

There are many levels and alternatives for intervention to meet the psychological reactions and psychopathology associated with AIDS. One level is volunteer organizations and support groups. Psychiatrists and other mental health professionals can provide services in hospitals, out-patient clinics, and private offices.

Crisis intervention may be indicated at the time of diagnosis and whenever suicidal thoughts develop. Individual therapy may be directed toward treatment of specific psychiatric problems, such as affective adjustment and anxiety disorders. Finally, psychotropic medications may be effective as adjuncts to therapy when they are indicated for the psychiatric problems that have developed. Special attention needs to be given to the physical condition of the patient, especially respiratory disorders, and liver impairment may contraindicate some types of medication. For example, use of benzodiazepines is contraindicated because of their depressive potential and because they may worsen the neurological impairment caused by HIV.

Thoughts of suicide ideation may occur at any time in relation to the development of AIDS. Health care givers must be alert to the need to take a suicide history, recognize and treat depression and organic brain syndrome, and provide continuous observation when indicated.

Many AIDS patients have central nervous system complications and a significant number of these patients manifest clinical symptoms. These complications may occur prior to any other manifestations of infection, and the complications increase with time. The first symptoms of central nervous system impairment may be behavioral disturbances, including agitation, depression, apathy, socially inappropriate behavior, hallucinations, delusions, anxiety, and memory impairment. A variety of organic mental syndromes have been observed in HIV-infected patients, including dementia, delirium, and organic personality syndrome. A common dysfunction is subacute encephalitis, which can present itself as a delirium, a mental disorder, or depression. The syndrome progresses over time to a severe chronic encephalopathy characterized by dementia, seizures, and death.

The dementia caused by encephalopathy associated with HIV infection is an organic brain syndrome. It is characterized by a loss of intellectual abilities that is sufficiently severe to interfere with the individual's social and occupational functioning. Congenitive functions that are impaired include memory, judgment, and abstract thinking. Other disturbances of higher cortical function include aphasia (disorder of language due to brain dysfunction), apraxia (inability to carry out motor activities), and agnosia (failure to recognize or identify objects). Personality changes include alteration of the characteristic personality or accentuation of personality traits. Loss of cortical inhibitions may lead to assaultive behavior or lack of social amenities. Other features include depression, psychosis, and anxiety. Therapy appropriate for dementia is primarily supportive, although haloperidol may reduce anxiety and agitation as well as psychotic symptomatology.

The psychiatric disorders associated with AIDS require not only the care and services of a physician in primary care internal medicine, but also physicians and health care personnel in psychiatry and mental health. Nursing care requirements will vary. The impairments associated with AIDS may also create the need to consider commitment to a mental health facility or utilization of guardianship proceedings. Either in-patient or out-patient placements may be appropriate.

1. Civil Commitments

Civil commitment is the exercise of the state's power to detain, institutionalize, and treat mentally ill persons. While commitment criteria vary from state to state, most states have adopted standards for commitment that employ two elements. First, all states require that an individual must be found mentally ill as determined by medical authorities. Unfortunately, mental illness is not defined in many states. Some states define mental illness circularly as being a condition for which there is a need for treatment. A typical statutory definition is provided in Missouri, which defines mental illness as a "state of impaired mental process, which impairment results in a distortion of a person's capacity to recognize reality due to hallucinations, delusions, faulty perceptions, or alterations of mood, and interferes with an individual's ability to reason, understand, or exercise control over his actions."

The second element varies in form and scope from state to state. Most states allow commitment upon a showing that an individual is dangerous. For instance, in California, a person may be certified for a 180–day commitment period if "[t]he person had attempted or inflicted physical harm upon the person of another, that act having resulted in his or her being taken into custody, and who presents, as a result of mental disorder or mental defect, a demonstrated danger of inflicting substantial physical harm upon others." Some states require that dangerousness be established by a recent overt act or threat.

A few states allow commitment of those who are gravely disabled or are unable to provide for their basic needs. Several states do not use the term "gravely disabled" when setting forth substantial commitment criteria. Instead, they list descriptions of conditions that are equivalent to a standard of "grave disability." Florida, for example, permits commitment of a person if "[h]e is manifestly incapable of surviving alone or with the help of willing and responsible family or friends, including available alternative services, and, without treatment, he or she is likely to suffer from neglect or refusal to care for himself, and such neglect or refusal poses a real and present threat of substantial harm to his well-being." Illinois permits commitment of a "person who is mentally ill and who because of his illness is unable to provide for his basic needs so as to guard himself from serious harm." Finally, some states, such as New York, merely require a showing that an individual is in need of treatment.

Many states require that the "least restrictive" or "least drastic" treatment alternative be imposed. Under this standard a court may order hospitalization only if the person meets the commitment criteria and if hospitalization is the least drastic form of treatment available.

Some persons subject to civil commitment who have AIDS may be subject to commitment independent of their AIDS diagnosis. In *Matter of Commitment of B.S.*, the patient suffered from organic brain damage resulting partly from drug abuse, partly from a period of hypoxia occurring during a hospital procedure, and partly from AIDS. When not medicated, she was often violent, hitting and biting nurses, wandering the corridors, and getting into bed with other patients. In upholding the patient's commitment, the New Jersey appellate court did not find it necessary to deal with the question of whether a mentally ill person should be committed because of an inability to appreciate the dangers associated with an AIDS condition. The court found that the patient qualified for commitment without regard to her AIDS condition because she was unable to care for herself as the result of her mental condition.

The psychological and psychiatric effects of HIV infection will in some cases provide a basis for a finding of mental illness. The behavioral effects of HIV infection also may meet the standard for commitment. In most HIV cases in which commitment is appropriate, it is likely that a finding that the patient is gravely disabled or is unable to provide for his or her basic needs will serve as the basis for commitment. However, it is likely that in most cases involving HIV-infected patients, an alternative that is less restrictive than involuntary hospitalization will be appropriate.

2. Guardianship

As a result of mental impairment caused by HIV infection, a person may need to have a guardian or a conservator appointed. A guardianship protects a disabled person by appointing a guardian to make personal decisions for the ward or to make decisions concerning the ward's estate. Guardianship proceedings require a showing that the individual is unable to manage his or her personal affairs or financial matters.

A guardian of the estate is appointed to manage the ward's financial matters to the extent that the ward is incapable of doing so. If the ward's assets are modest, a domestic partner, family member, or a public agency may be appointed. Where the assets are substantial, a bank may be appointed. A guardian of the person makes decisions concerning living arrangements, consent for medical treatment, and other personal decisions.

Guardianship procedures vary from state to state. Notice to the alleged disabled person must be served, including a copy of the petition and summons to the court hearing. Most states provide the right to a jury trial if the allegedly disabled person opposes the guardianship. At the court hearing, the petitioner presents evidence that the alleged disabled person is in need of a guardian of the person, the estate, or both. The defense may call witnesses, including physicians and health care personnel to testify as expert witnesses.

Formerly, a finding of a need for guardianship deprived the ward of all decisionmaking powers. More recently, guardianships have been tailored to the disability of the individual. Many states provide that a guardianship may be ordered only to the extent necessitated by the individual's actual mental, physical, and adaptive limitations. Most HIV-infected persons who require guardianships will qualify for a limited guardianship to meet the specific needs created by the mental impairment caused by the HIV infection.

The mental impairments caused by HIV infection in some persons may qualify them for federally-supported vocational rehabilitation and services to facilitate independent living. Vocational rehabilitation services are provided to "handicapped" persons, including any person who, by reason of physical or mental disability, is substantially handicapped with respect to employment and who can reasonably be expected to benefit from the services that are provided. Federal legislation bestows legal rights, such as a right to independent living to handicapped persons. A program to provide independent living conditions for unemployable handicapped persons is provided by federal law. Federal law also establishes funding for state programs designed to provide comprehensive services to severely handicapped persons who do not have employment potential in order to help place them in independent living situations in the community. In *Doe v. Centinela Hospital*, a federal district court in California found HIV infection to constitute a handicap that precluded discrimination against otherwise qualified individuals.

CHAPTER VIII

INTERNATIONAL LAW

A. INTRODUCTION

Although a few totalitarian governments continue
for political reasons to claim otherwise, it generally
is accepted that AIDS now has established an impressive foothold in every country in the world.
This fact has made the need for global cooperation
very important and has resulted in the establishment of both bilateral and multilateral research and
information programs. Nevertheless, the rights of
persons with AIDS to engage in travel, to enter or
remain in a given country temporarily to obtain
medical attention, and to permanently relocate
across national borders is governed by domestic
rather than international law. Similarly, the task
of protecting HIV-infected individuals from unwarranted discrimination has been left to national
courts and legislatures. The result has been a
disjointed system in which persons with AIDS often
suffer greatly with little or no hope of effective legal
redress.

B. ROLE OF INTERNATIONAL LAW

1. Definition

At one time, international law was defined as that body of legal principles that governed the relationships between and among countries. Under this definition, only countries were subject to international law and only they had rights and duties under it. Because individuals were thought to be beyond the reach of international law, many early writers referred to international law as the law of nations. The two terms are now considered fungible, although few modern commentators use the phrase "law of nations" except when describing historical matters.

In the period since 1945, international law has enjoyed unprecedented growth in both recognition and importance due to the belief that only through a strengthening of international law can world conflict be avoided. As such, the old definition of international law is no longer accurate and has been discarded. In its place, a completely different definition has been developed. Under contemporary standards, international law is said to consist of that body of law that governs countries and that cannot be lawfully changed or ignored by individual countries. Put another way, international law is that law to which all countries must conform their policies, practices, and domestic law.

2. Terminology

Before attempting to determine the exact parameters of modern international law and describing the enforcement mechanisms that exist to deal with its violation, it is necessary to take note of the problem of jargon. There are several terms that have unique meanings in the field of international law. First, international law refers to countries as states. This can be very confusing, since countries that are based on a federal union model, such as the United States, use the term "states" to refer to the individual jurisdictions within the union. Second, international law uses the term municipal law when speaking of the law of a given country. It should be noted that the term "municipal law" is considered outdated by many commentators and is rapidly being replaced by the term domestic law.

Third, international law often is divided into subcategories known as public international law and private international law. While this distinction is without legal significance, it provides a convenient way of referring to the two main branches of international law. Public international law refers to traditional international law matters, such as the making of treaties and the exchanging of ambassadors. Private international law refers to the legal aspects of trade and commerce between individuals from different countries. In most instances, use of the term international law knowingly or unknowingly refers to public international law.

Fourth, international law often is confused with the fields of foreign law and comparative law. In fact, international, foreign, and comparative law are all distinct areas of law. The term foreign law is used with respect to the study of the law of a third country. Thus, for example, an American lawyer might refer to the law of Japan as foreign law, to distinguish it from the law of the United States. In contrast, comparative law refers to the field of law that compares the legal systems of different countries. An examination of how rapists are treated by the United States legal system, as opposed to the legal system of Canada, is an example of comparative law.

Fifth, international law can, but usually does not, refer to the law applicable to international organizations such as the United Nations and the International Red Cross. Depending upon the particular circumstances that are present, such organizations may be governed by domestic law, international law, or their own internal law. When no particular international organization is being discussed, this body of law is referred to as international organizations law. If, however, a particular international organization is being mentioned, it is common to use the name of the organization. Thus, one speaks of United Nations Law and European Community Law. Finally, international law must be distinguished from the law of conflicts. The law of conflicts is that body of domestic law that determines, in case of a conflict, which jurisdiction's law is to be applied. A conflict may arise because the plaintiff and defendant are from different countries or because they are from the same country but different parts.

3. Content

As a practical matter, the content of international law consists of the treaties that have been entered into by states, the resolutions that have been promulgated by international organizations, and the decisions that have been issued by international tribunals. Because international law is not yet as well developed as domestic law, the writings of international law scholars, the principles contained in the natural law, and what is referred to as customary international law also contribute to the body of international law. Needless to say, determining the content of international law is an often frustrating and difficult enterprise.

In the view of some commentators, unless a treaty exists that authoritatively regulates a matter, international law can do no more than provide a suggested solution to a specific question. Scholars who take this view assert that in the absence of a clear decision to bind itself to a particular rule or norm of conduct, all countries are free to do as they wish. Proponents of this view argue that all countries possess an inherent right of sovereignty and self-determination that cannot be limited except by the country itself. Of course, even the most ardent adherents of this position recognize the practical reality that a country's neighbors may try to prevent a particular course of action by the use of military force, the imposition of economic sanctions, or by appeals to the consciences of the country's leaders.

In contrast, other scholars assert that there is a body of non-consensual law that limits the rights of countries (and their leaders) from acting as they please. This body is referred to at different times by the terms natural law, *jus cogens*, and general principles of law. While each of these terms has precise meanings and refers to a slightly different aspect of the concept, it will suffice here to remain focused on the basic idea that all three have in common. Scholars who believe in the existence of non-consensual law (so named because it does not depend on the consent of a particular country before that country becomes bound) suggest that there are certain rights that are so fundamental to human beings that no country may legally violate, diminish, or terminate them. There is sharp disagreement, however, as to exactly what rights are included in the definition of fundamental rights, despite the fact that there are dozens of international treaties, conventions, and proclamations that expressly recognize specific rights in individuals.

4. Enforcement Mechanisms

At the heart of the international legal system is the United Nation's International Court of Justice (ICJ). The ICJ is often referred to as the World Court, although in reality its jurisdiction is much more limited. The ICJ was founded in 1945 and continues the work of the Permanent Court of International Justice, which was established in 1920 under the auspices of the League of Nations. All countries that are members of the UN automatically become parties to the Statute of the ICJ. The Statute of the ICJ serves as the court's constitution. Countries that are not members of the UN may become parties to the Statute of the ICJ by meeting the conditions that the UN has set for such countries.

The ICJ is made up of fifteen judges, no two of whom may come from the same country. They are elected by the UN to nine year terms and are eligible for re-election. Although judges may come from any country, in practice there always is a judge from each of the five countries that are permanent members of the UN Security Council (China, France, Great Britain, Russia, and the United States). The permanent seat of the ICJ is located at The Hague in the Netherlands.

Although it is called the World Court, the ICJ can only hear suits between countries. Thus, individuals who have grievances against a country (be it their own country or that of a foreign country) have no standing before the ICJ. Even where they are able to convince a country to take on their claim, it has been held by the ICJ that the case will be dismissed if it is shown that there is an "absence of any bond of attachment" between the country bringing the case and the individual for whom the claim is asserted. As a practical matter, it has been very difficult for individuals to convince countries to bring claims on their behalf before the ICJ.

While all countries that are members of the UN are parties to the Statute of the ICJ, only a handful of countries have agreed without reservation to the jurisdiction of the ICJ. In most instances, countries have deposited reservations indicating what kinds of suits they will allow the ICJ to hear. The ability of countries to unilaterally limit the jurisdiction of the ICJ and the widespread use of this option, has left the ICJ rather impotent.

Even where countries have not deposited reservations, the ICJ has no power to force a country to obey its decisions. When, in 1980, the ICJ, acting on a complaint filed by the United States, entered a final judgment ordering Iran to immediately release the hostages it had been holding in the United States Embassy in Tehran for more than six months, Iran took the position that the ICJ's order was without legal force. Although final judgments of the ICJ technically can be enforced by the UN Security Council, in reality the ICJ depends entirely upon voluntary compliance with its orders. In the case of the hostages, the ICJ's order had no effect. The hostages remained in captivity for eight more months and were finally freed only after Iran decided to enter into a complex arrangement with the United States, using Algeria as an intermediary in the protracted negotiations.

In addition to the ICJ, four other international courts exist: the Court of Justice of the European Communities, the European Court of Human Rights, the Benelux Court of Justice, and the Inter–American Court of Human Rights. These courts have the potential to become very important sources of individual rights. The European Court of Human Rights has begun to have a significant impact on civil liberties, and has started to receive AIDS cases. In *Demai v. France,* for example, the court was asked to hear a case involving a French citizen who had contracted HIV during a blood transfusion. Before the court could issue a final ruling, however, the parties settled. Nevertheless, the ultimate potential impact of these courts is limited by the fact that they are regional institutions lacking the universal character of the ICJ. The decisions of the Court of Justice of the European Communities, for example, affect only those countries that are members of the Communities. The European Court of Human Rights touches only those nations included in the Council of Europe. The Benelux Court of Justice is limited to Belgium, the Netherlands, and Luxembourg. Finally, the Inter–American Court of Human Rights is of relevance only to those countries of the Americas that are parties to the American Convention on Human Rights. It should be noted that the United States is not a party to the American Convention on Human Rights.

Because of the limitations of the existing international courts, there has been an on-going attempt to persuade domestic courts to enforce international law rights. For the most part, this attempt has been unsuccessful. When faced with an argument based on international law, domestic courts have typically taken the position that international law is subordinate to domestic law. Even when faced with a specific international instrument that contains clearly-delineated "rights," domestic courts have held that the instruments are merely aspirational and their language precatory. *Jamur Productions Corp. v. Quill.*

5. AIDS and International Law

As noted above, it currently is not possible as a practical matter to sue on claims founded on international law on behalf of individuals; this may change in the future. Even if it does not, it is possible that in a given case a reference to international law might prove helpful. Because of their global character, the instruments of the UN that recognize that individuals have specific legal rights that cannot be taken away by any government are worthy of extended discussion.

The UN Charter, which is modelled after the constitution of the United States, provides in Article 55 that the UN should promote, and all countries should respect, the fundamental rights of individuals regardless of their race, sex, language, or religion. Shortly after promulgation of the UN Charter, a Universal Declaration of Human Rights was unanimously enacted by the UN General Assembly.

Article 1 of the Universal Declaration states that all persons are born free and equal in dignity and rights. Article 2 underscores this by stating that no one is to be discriminated against by reason of their race, color, sex, language, religion, political opinion, national or social origin, property, birth, or other status.

For purposes of AIDS advocacy, Article 2 is an important tool. Because of its instruction that persons are not to be discriminated against because of their "status," the reach of Article 2, and thus of the Universal Declaration, goes further than that of Article 55 of the UN Charter, which identifies only the characteristics of race, sex, language, and religion as improper bases of discrimination. The Universal Declaration has several other articles that also speak to AIDS issues. Article 7 states that all persons are equal before the law and cannot be discriminated against by the law. Article 9 states that no one may be exiled in an arbitrary fashion, while Article 12 extends to all persons the right to be free from arbitrary interferences with their privacy. Article 13(2) ensures the right to travel across national borders.

In unison, these articles provide a powerful command to nations that they respect the privacy of persons with AIDS. In addition, Articles 9 and 13 clearly prohibit countries from either advocating or implementing programs to keep persons with AIDS out of their territory or confining them to remote quarantine centers.

The most important articles, however, are Articles 21(2), 23(1), and 25(1). Article 21(2) states that everyone has the right of equal access to public service in his or her own country. Article 23(1) extends the right to work and to be free from unemployment to all people. Finally, Article 25(1) states that all people have the right to a standard of living adequate for the health and well-being of themselves and their families, including food, clothing, housing, medical care, and necessary social services. Moreover, Article 25(1) states that all persons have the right to security in the event that they are unable to provide for themselves due to "circumstances beyond his control." Taken together, Articles 21(2), 23(1), and 25(1) can easily be read as requiring nations to ensure that persons with AIDS are not discriminated against in the workplace, obtain adequate medical care, and have a fair share of public funds allocated for AIDS research.

C. UNITED STATES IMMIGRATION LAW

Because of the current state of international law, the legal problems faced by people with AIDS must be addressed through domestic legal systems. One key area that has received extensive attention is the rights of such individuals to engage in international travel and to relocate from one country to another, either on a temporary or permanent basis. Because the United States has had a highly visible role in these matters, a review of its policies provides useful insight on the principal considerations that come into play whenever people with AIDS seek to travel across national borders.

1. Basic Statutory Framework

United States immigration policy is contained in two key pieces of legislation: the Immigration and Nationality Act of 1952 (INA) and the Immigration

Reform and Control Act of 1986 (IRCA). Although other statutes, such as the Immigration Act of 1990, also come into play, the INA and the IRCA provide the basic statutory framework of American immigration policy.

The INA and IRCA have been enacted pursuant to Congress' perceived power to exclusively regulate immigration. Although Article 1, section 8, clause 4 of the United States Constitution provides that Congress has the power to establish a "uniform Rule of Naturalization," the Constitution is silent with respect to Congress' power to regulate the admission and expulsion of aliens. In a long line of cases, however, the United States Supreme Court has held, based on a combination of international and constitutional law principles, that Congress also enjoys the exclusive power to control immigration. Because of these cases, no state may pass or attempt to enforce legislation that affects immigration or naturalization matters.

Responsibility for immigration matters is divided among the United States Departments of State, Justice, Labor, and Health and Human Services. The State Department is responsible for issuing immigrant visas. Any alien who wishes to enter the United States must obtain a visa indicating that they have been found eligible to enter the United States. There are many different types of visas, although all visas fall into one of two categories: those that are subject to numerical limits and those that are not. A very typical sort of visa is the B–2 tourist visa. Aliens who wish to visit the United

States for short periods of time (such as while traveling on vacation) must obtain a B–2 visa from the United States embassy or consulate located in their home country. Embassies and consulates are the responsibility of the State Department and are staffed by State Department employees.

The Justice Department plays the largest role in immigration matters. Although the Attorney General, as the nation's chief federal law enforcement officer, is clothed with the duty of administering the nation's immigration laws, it is the Immigration and Naturalization Service (INS) that operates the immigration laws on a day-to-day basis. The INS is a part of the Justice Department and is headed by a Commissioner, who is appointed by the President on the recommendation of the Attorney General. Below the Commissioner are Regional Commissioners and below them some three dozen district directors.

The INS is one leg of what collectively is known as the Executive Office of Immigration Review (EOIR). In addition to the INS, the EOIR is made up of the immigration courts and the Board of Immigration Appeals (BIA). Both the immigration courts and the BIA are part of the Justice Department and report to the Associate Attorney General in charge of the EOIR and, in turn, to the Attorney General. Decisions of the immigration courts, whose judges are known as special inquiry officers, go to the BIA, whose five members are appointed by the Attorney General. Certain decisions of the BIA are reviewable by the Attorney General, while certain final orders of the BIA can be contested in the federal courts.

Aliens who enter the country with the intention of applying for employment will at some point come into contact with the Labor Department, which is responsible for determining which aliens may lawfully obtain work and for issuing certificates to those who qualify. In this regard, the Labor Department works closely with the employment service office in the state in which the alien seeks to be employed.

In the AIDS context, the most important federal department concerned with the administration of the immigration laws is the Department of Health and Human Services. The PHS, which is part of the Department, is responsible for determining whether a particular alien is medically fit to enter the United States. To accomplish this task, the PHS has stationed doctors throughout the world and at various ports of entry in this country. An alien who is found to be medically unfit will not be allowed to enter the United States for two reasons. First, there is a concern that aliens who are medically unfit will, if admitted, further tax the already overextended American health care system. Second, in the case of contagious conditions such as AIDS, there is a fear that an unhealthy alien will spread his or her condition to American citizens.

2. Classification of HIV as a Dangerous Contagious Disease

Throughout its history, the United States has sought to exclude certain types of aliens thought to pose special risks. Currently, the INA lists thirty-three types of aliens who are to be excluded. These categories are very comprehensive and include beggars, polygamists, prostitutes, stowaways, drug users, illiterates, anarchists, and Nazi war criminals. There also is a category for those aliens "who are afflicted with any dangerous contagious disease." 8 U.S.C.A. § 1182(a)(6).

Because the INA does not define what diseases are to be considered "dangerous contagious disease[s]," it has fallen to the PHS to make the decision. By the beginning of the 1980s (that is, immediately before AIDS was first recognized), the PHS had identified seven diseases as being dangerous contagious diseases: chancroid, gonorrhea, granuloma inguinale, leprosy, lymphogranuloma venereum, syphilis, and tuberculosis.

In 1986, the PHS recommended for the first time that AIDS be added to the list. A Notice of Proposed Rulemaking was therefore issued so that the formal process of amending the list could begin. 51 Fed. Reg. 15,354 (1986). In support of its decision, the PHS argued that it was inconsistent to have chancroid and lymphogranuloma venereum, two highly infectious venereal diseases, on the list while AIDS was not on the list.

In the following year, three events took place that propelled AIDS onto the list. First, President Reagan announced his support for the proposed rule and called for the immediate testing of all immigrants to the United States. Second, Congress, spurred on by Senator Jesse Helms, approved an amendment to a supplemental appropriations bill that required AIDS to be added to the list. Finally, the PHS, having finished its public review period, concluded that despite the protests that had been raised during the public review, the proposed rule should be finalized. Accordingly, a final rule was issued adding AIDS to the list. 52 Fed. Reg. 21,532 (1987). Subsequently, the rule was withdrawn and replaced with a final rule that substituted the term HIV for the term AIDS. 52 Fed. Reg. 32,541 (1987). As a result of this substitution, it did not matter whether an alien showed symptoms of having AIDS. All that was required was that the alien test positive for HIV infection.

The decision to classify HIV as a dangerous contagious disease has had little practical effect: in any given year, only a few hundred aliens are excluded from the United States based on their HIV status. Nevertheless, the mere existence of the ban has prompted gay and lesbian groups, AIDS activists, and others, including the American Bar Association, to condemn the decision as a particularly offensive example of government insensitivity to and harassment of persons with AIDS. Along similar lines, numerous international organizations, including the International Red Cross and the International

Planned Parenthood Federation, have criticized the decision and have from time to time boycotted or threatened to boycott AIDS meetings held in the United States. In 1991, for example, Harvard University had to move the site of the Eighth International Conference on AIDS from Boston to Amsterdam after England announced that it intended to boycott the gathering to protest the United States' immigration policies.

In 1990, the United States General Accounting Office issued an opinion that the supplemental appropriations legislation passed by Congress that had obligated President Reagan to add AIDS to the PHS list of dangerous contagious diseases was a "one-time action" that was intended "to compel the immediate issuance of regulations, not to mandate the indefinite maintenance of regulations." As a result, during the 1992 presidential election Bill Clinton pledged to remove HIV from the PHS list. Shortly after the election, however, Congress passed legislation that attached a permanent HIV-immigrant ban to a bill providing AIDS funding to the National Institutes of Health.

The current ban is subject to certain exceptions and loopholes. For example, most short-term visitors (as opposed to those seeking more permanent immigrant or refugee status) are able to enter and leave the United States without having to submit to testing. Moreover, the government can lift the ban on a case-by-case. In 1994, Attorney General Janet Reno granted a ten-day waiver of the ban to all HIV-infected individuals participating in Gay

Games IV, an international sports competition being held in New York City. Where exceptions are made, however, neither the State Department nor the INS guarantees confidentiality in the handling of AIDS-related information.

D. GLOBAL EFFORTS

AIDS has been the subject of government action in many countries. At the same time, a number of international organizations have undertaken AIDS-related programs and initiatives.

1. Foreign Countries

The response to AIDS in countries other than the United States has ranged from reasonable to illogical. During the early years of the epidemic, many countries, including Australia, Britain, and Sweden, enacted or considered quarantine proposals as a means of dealing with AIDS. Only Cuba, however, actually carried out widespread isolation. Between 1986 and 1993, persons found to be HIV-positive were taken into custody and placed in state-run institutions known as "sanatorios." The enormous cost of running these facilities, coupled with the deterioration of the Cuban economy following the collapse of the Soviet Union, eventually forced the government to abandon its efforts.

The early years of the epidemic also saw many countries take the view that AIDS could be contained by limiting the contact that their citizens had with foreigners. In the city of Klagenfurt,

Austria, for example, an attempt was made to refuse work permits to foreigners who could not prove that they were HIV-negative. In the state of Bavaria in Germany, a law requiring certain foreigners to submit to HIV screening tests was passed. A short time later, an American citizen was sentenced to two years in prison for having practiced unsafe sex after he learned that he had AIDS. In Bangladesh, the government at one point considered banning the importation of used clothes from the United States for fear that the clothes might spread AIDS. In Japan, there remains a lingering belief among some members of the public that AIDS can be transmitted by foreigners through the sharing of swimming pools and restrooms.

When the Chinese government learned that an American citizen in Beijing had AIDS, it ordered him to leave the country. Because the Chinese government would not allow him to fly out of China on a commercial jet, the United States government was forced to fly him out on a military medical evacuation plan. Similarly, during the annual Carnival in Rio de Janeiro, Brazilian health authorities at one point attempted to poll foreign visitors on their sexual preferences in an attempt to determine whether the Carnival was a time when AIDS was likely to enter the country. When the government was unable to get international airlines to cooperate with it and many tourist officials worried that visitors would shun the Carnival, the effort was dropped.

Today, most countries have come to recognize that AIDS is a global problem that cannot simply be shut out. In large part, this change in view has come about due to international medical statistics. As many as 7,500 new cases of HIV infection occur each day; 90% of these cases are located in countries in the developing world. At the end of 1995, 20 million people (including 1.5 million children) were thought to have contracted HIV. Of this number, 13 million were in Africa and 3.5 million were in Asia. The number of HIV cases is expected to grow to 40 million by the year 2000, with Asia likely to experience the largest increase (up to 9 million additional cases). Unlike the situation in the United States, 75% of worldwide HIV transmissions now occur by means of heterosexual intercourse. As a result, 14 million women are expected to be infected with HIV by the year 2000; by that time, 4 million women will have died from AIDS.

2. International Organizations

Because of the rapid spread of AIDS cases, numerous international organizations are now involved in the fight against AIDS. Chief among them is the World Health Organization (WHO), a specialized UN agency. It was created in 1948 to coordinate international health efforts and to replace what had become an unwieldy collection of other health organizations, such as the Office International d'Hygiene Publique, the Health Organization of the League of Nations, and the Pan–American Sanitary Organization.

In 1983, WHO, at its headquarters in Geneva, Switzerland, began reviewing the existing information on AIDS. In 1984, regional WHO meetings were organized in Europe and in the Americas. In 1985, WHO convened the first international congress on AIDS in Atlanta in cooperation with the CDC. Following the congress, a network of twenty-six WHO collaborating centers were established. In 1986, a second international congress on AIDS was held by WHO in Paris, followed by a third congress in 1987 in Washington, D.C. Since then, WHO has sponsored or co-sponsored numerous international AIDS conferences at various sites around the world, including an inter-government gathering in London in 1988. Many observers believe that the London conference was a critical turning point in the effort to gain widespread governmental agreement on the need to move aggressively against AIDS.

By the end of 1986, WHO's expanding role in the coordination of the international effort against AIDS required greater administrative expertise. As a result, WHO created a Special Programme on AIDS to bring together within one department all of its AIDS-related activities. The program's name subsequently was changed to the Global Programme on AIDS (GPA).

Between 1986 and 1995, the GPA was the world's preeminent AIDS organization. At its peak, it commanded a staff of nearly one hundred persons in Geneva and a budget in excess of $60 million. Although the GPA did not undertake any biomedical research on its own and funded only a small portion of the world's total AIDS research, its activities extended over a wide spectrum. It promoted the sharing of information through the holding of international meetings, suggested strategies for the care of persons suffering from AIDS, examined the interaction of AIDS with other forms of disease, such as malaria and tuberculosis, prepared guidelines for scientists engaged in AIDS drug and vaccine testing and trials, conducted global AIDS-education programs, served as a clearing house for AIDS information, and, beginning in 1988, annually promoted the observance of International AIDS Awareness Day on December 1.

One of the most important tasks carried out by the GPA was the establishment of an AIDS reporting system that tracked new medical cases of AIDS. In all, 176 countries joined the GPA's reporting network. The GPA also formulated a global strategy against AIDS that was subsequently endorsed by the World Health Assembly, the UN General Assembly, the UN Economic and Social Council (UN-ESCO), and the 1987 Venice summit of Western political leaders.

The GPA also worked closely with national and regional AIDS groups and experts. A total of 151 countries established national AIDS committees that worked with the GPA in formulating appropriate AIDS strategies for their countries. The GPA conferred with leading experts from around the world as well as with numerous agencies of the UN, including the World Bank, the International Labor Organization, UNICEF, and the World Tourism Organization. Finally, through its regional offices, such as the Pan–American Health Organization, WHO sponsored regional AIDS surveillance and tracking studies, medical and scientific conferences, and education programs.

Despite the importance of its mission and the acclaim that its activities received, the GPA attracted a fair amount of criticism. In 1990, Dr. Jonathan M. Mann, an American AIDS expert who had served as the director of the GPA since its creation, resigned following a highly public clash with Dr. Hiroshi Nakajima. Dr. Nakajima had become WHO's director-general in 1988 after a lengthy and highly political battle for the position. In the view of Dr. Mann, Dr. Nakajima had sought to use his position to direct financing and manpower away from the GPA in favor of non-AIDS programs. Although Dr. Nakajima contended that he fully supported the GPA and appointed Dr. Michael H. Merson, another American AIDS expert, to replace Dr. Mann, in 1994 it was announced that WHO planned to shut down the GPA during 1995.

On January 1, 1996, the GPA's activities were transferred to a new agency known as the United Nations inter-agency program on AIDS, or UN–AIDS. UN–AIDS, which is sponsored by a variety of UN entities, including UNESCO, UNICEF, the United Nations Family and Planning Agency, the World Bank, and WHO, is headed by Dr. Peter Piot, a Belgian scientist who had served as the GPA's chief of research. Although Dr. Piot has promised that UN–AIDS will be just as aggressive as the

GPA, and has announced that one of UN–AIDS' top priorities will be the hunt for an HIV vaccine. many fear that the agency's mandate to streamline the UN's AIDS budget will cause UN–AIDS to be much less effective than the GPA.

Although WHO and others have stressed the need for cooperation among AIDS researchers and the adoption of policies towards persons with AIDS that are based on sound medical judgment rather than public hysteria, their pleas have often been ignored. Two notable examples involve the battle over the discovery of the virus that causes AIDS and the struggle surrounding international travel by people with AIDS.

The theory that AIDS was caused by a virus was proved in 1983 when researchers at the Paris-based Pasteur Institute, working under the direction of Dr. Luc Montagnier, announced the discovery of a virus they called LAV. A short time later, researchers at the National Cancer Institute (NCI) in Bethesda, Maryland, led by Dr. Robert Gallo, announced the discovery of a virus they called HTLV–III.

Although LAV and HTLV–III were soon determined to be nearly identical, a bitter dispute developed between the Pasteur Institute and the NCI over which team of scientists had been the first to discover the AIDS virus. At stake was scientific prestige and the right to collect royalties from patents on AIDS blood tests that were expected to generate $5 million per year in the United States alone. When the two sides deadlocked over the question, the Pasteur Institute brought a lawsuit against the United States government. *Institut Pasteur v. United States*.

The dispute appeared to be settled in 1987, when French Prime Minister Jacques Chirac and President Ronald Reagan entered into an executive agreement. As part of the agreement, a new AIDS research foundation was established in Paris under the joint direction of the Pasteur Institute and the United States Department of Health and Human Services. In the wake of the agreement, Drs. Montagnier and Gallo were recognized as the co-discoverers of the AIDS virus and the term HIV replaced both LAV and HTLV–III.

In 1990, however, the validity of the agreement was called into question by reports that the United States had suppressed documents that proved, as the Pasteur Institute alleged in its lawsuit, that Dr. Gallo stole Dr. Montagnier's discovery. Although a subsequent preliminary investigation cleared Dr. Gallo, plans for a second inquiry were announced immediately after the records of the preliminary investigation were made public. As a result, in 1994 the United States agreed to give France a larger share of the royalties generated by the patents, thereby tacitly admitting Dr. Gallo's improper use of HIV samples obtained from the Pasteur Institute. A short time later, citing lack of federal funding, Dr. Gallo left the NCI and established his own laboratory.

The question of whether people with AIDS should be permitted to engage in international travel became a source of considerable public attention early in the history of AIDS. As noted earlier, many countries, including the United States, initially sought to keep out HIV-infected individuals in the mistaken belief that doing so would keep the disease at bay. They took this action despite the fact that in 1985 the WHO determined that policies such as testing international travelers for AIDS and requiring such travelers to carry with them medical certificates indicating that they had been tested and found not to be infected were unwarranted by existing conditions and unlikely to make a positive contribution to the fight against AIDS.

During the past five years, many countries (but not the United States) have reconsidered their policies and have opted to follow the WHO's recommendations. As a result, international travel is today easier for HIV-infected persons than it was in the early days of the epidemic. Among the countries that have recently adopted more lenient policies are Costa Rica, South Africa, and Thailand. Nevertheless, travel is still difficult for HIV-infected individuals in a number of countries, including China, Russia, Vietnam, and Indonesia, which in 1994 refused to allow Magic Johnson to enter the country to play in an exhibition basketball game.

*

INDEX

References are to Pages

†